Digital Planning and Custom Orthodontic Treatment

Digital Planning and Custom Orthodontic Treatment

Edited by

Dr. K. Hero Breuning
Orthodontist and Consultant

Prof. Chung H. Kau
University of Alabama, Birmingham, AL, USA

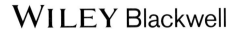

Registered Offices
John Wiley & Sons, Inc., 111 River Street, Hoboken, NJ 07030, USA
John Wiley & Sons, Ltd., The Atrium, Southern Gate, Chichester, West Sussex, PO19 8SQ, UK

Editorial Office
1606 Golden Aspen Drive, Suites 103 and 104, Ames, Iowa 50010, USA

For details of our global editorial offices, customer services, and more information about Wiley products visit us at www.wiley.com.

Wiley also publishes its books in a variety of electronic formats and by print-on-demand. Some content that appears in standard print versions of this book may not be available in other formats.

Library of Congress Cataloging-in-Publication Data

Names: Breuning, K. Hero, editor. | Kau, Chung How, editor.
Title: Digital planning and custom orthodontic treatment / edited by K. Hero Breuning, Chung H. Kau.
Description: Hoboken, NJ : John Wiley & Sons Inc., 2017. | Includes index.
Identifiers: LCCN 2016053363| ISBN 9781119087779 (pbk.) | ISBN 9781119087786 (Adobe PDF) | ISBN 9781119087793 (ePub)
Subjects: | MESH: Dental Impression Technique–instrumentation | Cone-Beam Computed Tomography–methods | Radiography, Dental, Digital–instrumentation
Classification: LCC RK521 | NLM WU 25 | DDC 617.6/43–dc23 LC record available at https://lccn.loc.gov/2016053363

Set in 10/12pt WarnockPro by Aptara Inc., New Delhi, India
Printed and bound in Singapore by Markono Print Media Pte Ltd

10 9 8 7 6 5 4 3 2 1

Contents

List of Contributors   *vii*
Preface   *xi*
Acknowledgments   *xv*

1   Documentation of the Dentition   *1*
K. Hero Breuning

2   Documentation of the Face   *9*
K. Hero Breuning

3   Dynamic Motion Capture of the Mandible   *15*
Shushu He and Chung H. Kau

4   Analysis of Digital Dental Documentation   *27*
K. Hero Breuning and Chung H. Kau

5   Orthodontic Treatment Planning   *31*
K. Hero Breuning and Chung H. Kau

6   Custom Appliance Design   *41*
K. Hero Breuning

7   Custom Appliance Fabrication and Transfer   *47*
K. Hero Breuning

8   Monitoring of Tooth Movement   *55*
Philippe Salah and K. Hero Breuning

9   Custom Retention after Orthodontic Treatment   *65*
K. Hero Breuning

10   The Invisalign System   *69*
Orhan Tuncay

11 Custom Lingual Appliances *81*
Neil Warshawsky, Thomas W. Örtendahl, Chung H. Kau and K. Hero Breuning

Appendix *115*

Index *117*

List of Contributors

K. Hero Breuning DDS, PhD

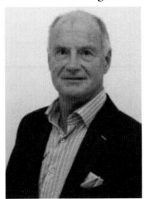

K. Hero Breuning studied dentistry and orthodontics at the University of Utrecht, the Netherlands and started a private orthodontic office in Tiel, the Netherlands. He worked closely together with maxillofacial surgeons and finished his PhD study on intraoral mandibular distraction at the Free University in Amsterdam. He was an assistant professor of 3D imaging at the Radboud University in Nijmegen, department of Orthodontics and Craniofacial Biology. He has published over 60 journal articles, lectured at major orthodontic meetings, and presented courses on various topics in 16 countries. He is a reviewer for several orthodontic journals. Currently he is a lecturer, researcher, consultant, and trainer in orthodontic offices. He loves his wife, children, and grandchildren and likes art, playing golf, skiing, and sailing.

Shushu He BDS, DDS, PhD

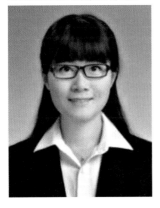

Shushu He studied at the West China School of Stomatology, Sichuan University, China and followed the Postgraduate program in Orthodontics at the Sichuan University, China. She was awarded as an Outstanding dental student and PhD student of Sichuan University and she was a visiting scholar at the University of Alabama at Birmingham, Alabama, USA. Currently she is a lecturer, at the State Key Laboratory of Oral Disease, Department of Orthodontics, West China School of Stomatology, Sichuan University, China. Shushu published several articles in peer-reviewed journals.

Chung H. Kau BDS, MScD, MBA, PhD, MOrth, FAMS, FDSGlas, FFD (Ortho), FDSEdin, FAMS, FICD

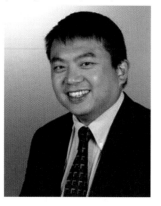

Chung H. Kau is Chairman and Professor at the Department of Orthodontics, University of Alabama at Birmingham, Alabama, USA. He is a Diplomate of the American Board of Orthodontics and enjoys practicing clinical orthodontics. He has a keen interest in three-dimensional and translational research. At present he is Principal Investigator on a number of grants and has a research involvement in excess of $3.2 million dollars. He actively contributes and publishes in the orthodontic literature and has over 300 peer-reviewed publications, conference papers, and lectures. He was also made the King James IV Professor by the Royal College of Surgeons in Edinburgh in 2011.

Thomas W. Örtendahl DDS

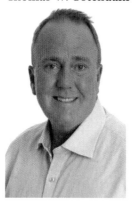

Thomas W. Örtendahl is a member of the Swedish Orthodontic Society, European Society, American Lingual Orthodontic Society, and the World Society of Lingual Orthodontics. He finished his dental training in 1983 at the University of Gothenburg, Sweden. In 1987, he finished his PhD studies and started his orthodontic training, which he completed in 1991. Since 1997, he has lectured worldwide on topics such as Esthetic Orthodontic treatment. He was a clinical instructor at the University of Gothenburg for 10 years. Dr. Örtendahl is co-author of the book *Lingual and Esthetic Orthodontics* (Quintessence Publishing, 2011) and is an adviser of several R & D departments. He is the head Orthodontist at the Smile Group, Mölndal, Sweden.

Philippe Salah PhD

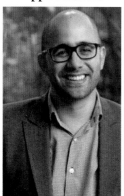

Philippe Salah graduated from École Polytechnique, Palaiseau, France with a PhD in Biophysics, and made orthodontics his favored research subject early in his career. In 2007, he co-founded the Harmony system, the first fully customized self-ligating lingual solution. Acquired in 2011 by American Orthodontics, Harmony experienced remarkable international growth. In 2013, animated by a passion for optimization and deep learning algorithms, he founded Dental Monitoring with a team of doctors, researchers, and engineers. Dental Monitoring is the world's first web and mobile application designed for self-monitoring dental treatment. It provides doctors with a live vision of their patient's treatment evolution that includes a very accurate 3D positioning of the teeth and effective communication and encouragement tools.

Orhan Tuncay DMD

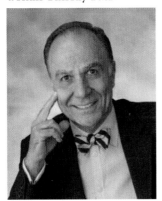

Philadelphia orthodontist Orhan Tuncay is an icon in the world of orthodontics. His academic career as an orthodontist is distinguished by his many contributions, innovations, and advances in the field of orthodontics. He has served as a department chairman for over 30 years and educated hundreds of orthodontists in the USA and abroad. His career started in the Department of Biochemistry at the University of Pennsylvania School of Dental Medicine. Subsequently, he received his orthodontic training at the same institution. He is known for his work on the biology of tooth movement, meta analyses, facial aesthetics, and 3D imaging and animation of the human face. He holds patents for his innovations in the field of 3D imaging. He has held innumerable official positions as an orthodontist in both scientific and professional organizations including: Chairman of the Council on Scientific Affairs of the American Association of Orthodontists, President of Greater Philadelphia Society of Orthodontists, and President of Craniofacial Biology Group of International & American Association for Dental Research. His textbook *The Invisalign® System* (Quintessence Publishing, 2006) is the first textbook in the world on Invisalign. Additionally, he is the founding editor of four international journals.

Neil Warshawsky DDS, MS

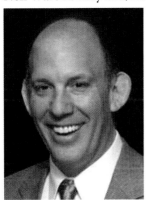

Neil Warshawsky is the founder and owner of Get It Straight Orthodontics, a leading orthodontic network in the Chicago area. A double board certified orthodontic specialist since 1992, he has over 23 years of experience with cleft palate and craniofacial cases. Currently, he is an Associate Professor of Surgery at the University of Illinois Craniofacial Center. In his private practice, he concentrates on esthetics and is one of largest volume users of Incognito™ lingual braces in the USA. He teaches advanced mechanical courses for 3M Oral Healthcare in North America as well as hands-on courses for Dentsply Raintree Essix around the world on Essix appliance fabrication and design. When he is not at work, he is an assistant scoutmaster for his sons' boy scout troop, at home with his high-school sweetheart, fishing at the family cabin with one of their three kids, or just out for a run.

Preface

The innovations in the documentation, analysis of a dental malocclusion, treatment planning, design, and fabrication of orthodontic appliances in the last decade have been major. The traditional method to document an orthodontic case with a plaster cast and two-dimensional (2D) images, and treat the patient with a selection of standard orthodontic brackets, after manual bracket placement with a set of standard and manually bended orthodontic wires, will not lead to the most efficient and controlled orthodontic treatment. Traditional appliances and mechanics will need more treatment time and the treatment result depends on the individual skills of the orthodontist. Currently, an orthodontist can use three-dimensional (3D) images for each patient who needs orthodontic and/or surgical treatment. Imaging of the dentition, skeleton, and the face in three dimensions allows a treatment plan to be made in 3D, and computer-aided design (CAD) and computer-aided manufacturing (CAM) to make customized orthodontic appliances (custom brackets, customized or custom aligners) to be used for the orthodontic treatment. If these custom appliances are used, increased efficiency and control during orthodontic treatment can be expected. CAD/CAM procedures can replace the "art" of bracket selection, bracket positioning, and manual wire bending.

Patients now demand to see and discuss diagnostic setups of the dentition and the prediction of facial changes caused by orthodontic and maxillofacial treatment before the start of treatment. They also wish to be treated in less time, with less visible appliances without the need for extensive cooperation during treatment. They should get relevant information from the monitoring of the speed of tooth movement into the planned direction during treatment. If tooth movement does not proceed as planned (because of appliance failures or inefficient mechanics), an alert should be sent to both the orthodontist and the patient. If skeletal correction during orthodontic treatment is indicated, this surgery should be an integrated part of the treatment planning and the actual treatment.

Virtual treatment planning in 3D of both the dentition and the skeletal changes will allow prediction of the facial changes after treatment. Because accurate dental and virtual surgical planning is now possible, even the amount of tooth movement needed before and after surgery can be predicted and evaluated

If required, maxillofacial surgery can be performed at an earlier time during orthodontic treatment, probably even after the initial correction of the dentition. Early surgical correction ("surgery first") can be indicated to correct the facial aesthetics and oral functions of the patient as soon as possible. Because virtual planning on 3D images with a 1 : 1 ratio is used, maxillofacial surgery can be more predictable and controlled.

The orthodontist and maxillofacial surgeon could send the 3D documentation and treatment plan to a dental or surgical lab for segmentation of the dentition and parts of the skull to make an initial setup. After segmentation of the dentition, the dental lab technician can make an initial simulation of the treatment planned by the dental specialist or maxillofacial surgeon. But the dental professional or maxillofacial surgeon can also perform this segmentation process and simulation (setup) in their own office with dedicated software programs. If the lab has made the initial setup, an orthodontist needs to make a definitive setup with CAD/CAM software. Before the introduction of the planned treatment and alternatives for this treatment, a setup can be discussed with other dental professionals.

Digital documentation in 3D with a ratio of 1 : 1 and digital dental and skeletal setups are required to design and fabricate orthodontic and surgical appliances. Introduction of the actual situation and the planned treatment with the use of a "virtual head" will be the most reliable way to show and discuss the planned treatment with the patient.

After acceptance of the treatment plan and its costs, custom orthodontic and surgical appliances used for this treatment can be designed. Removable appliances, fixed appliances and a set of aligners or a combination of these appliances can be used for orthodontic treatment. Usually, a dental lab will design the selected appliance systems (CAD). The orthodontist should approve the design of the appliances (e.g. the bracket position or the position of the attachments for aligner treatment), and then these appliances (including a set of custom bend arch wires for fixed appliance treatment) should be fabricated for effective and controlled tooth movement. For transfer of the planned bracket or attachment position on the final setup to the actual dentition of the patient, indirect bonding procedures are needed. Because patients ask to reduce treatment time with fixed appliances, treatment can be started with fixed custom orthodontic appliance systems and finished with clear aligners.

This "hybrid" orthodontic treatment approach (orthodontic treatment with a combination of appliances) will be the treatment of choice in the near future. Only increased control of all treatment procedures and the monitoring of treatment changes will enable treatment of an increasing amount of patients in a more predictable, more effective way without reduction of the quality of the treatment outcome. Both patients and referring dentists will appreciate the planning of the dental and surgical treatment on a virtual head and will love to see the prediction of the dental and facial outcome before the start of treatment.

The monitoring of tooth movement with intra-oral scans and intra-oral pictures taken at planned intervals will allow the planned treatment to be planned and optimized.

In this book, an overview of new developments in orthodontics—with an emphasis on 3D imaging, the digital planning of treatment, the CAD/CAM fabrication of appliances, and the monitoring of treatment during and after treatment—will be presented. The workflow for several custom appliance systems (Invisalign, Incognito, Harmony, Insignia, eBrace/eLock, and suresmile) will be introduced by experienced users of these systems. Recent improvements of custom systems will be presented in each chapter.

The content of this book will change in the years to come, so there will be a need for an update of the published information in the future.

For a full list of the companies who have kindly allowed us to use their images, please see the appendix at the back of the book.

The book's eleven chapters reflect a patient's workflow:

Chapter 1: Documentation of the Dentition
Chapter 2: Documentation of the Face

Chapter 3: Dynamic Motion Capture of the Mandible

Chapter 4: Analysis of the Documentation

Chapter 5: Treatment Planning

Chapter 6: Custom Appliance Design

Chapter 7: Custom Appliance Fabrication and Transfer to the Dentition

Chapter 8: Monitoring of Treatment

Chapter 9: Retention of Treatment

Chapter 10: Aligners (The Invisalign System)

Chapter 11: Custom Lingual Appliances

K. Hero Breuning and Chung H. Kau

Acknowledgments

K. Hero Breuning would like to thank Professor Anne Marie Kuijpers-Jagtman, because she allowed him to explore the new developments in orthodontics. Of course, he was very happy that Professor Chung H. Kau became interested in the project to write a book to show the new developments in orthodontics. Together, we introduced the COT system (Customized Orthodontic Treatment) as a concept. Both Anne Marie and Chung How recognized that the digital planning of orthodontic treatment and the use of customized appliances will become an alternative to traditional impressions of the dentition, 2D radiographs, digital 2D photographs, and setups of the dentition with plaster and wax. I am very grateful to publish the chapters written by the co-authors. They have shared their knowledge with us and the reader. And I would like to thank the companies who took their time to share their newest developments with me and allowed us to publish some of their images. Finally I would like to thank the editors working at Wiley for all their hard work in translating the English of a non-native speaker into readable English.

Chung H. Kau also thanks the authors of the chapters and the editor for their excellent work and of course the companies who allowed publication of the images used in this book.

1

Documentation of the Dentition

K. Hero Breuning

Introduction

There is a growing demand for innovative ways to record the dentition and craniofacial complex. New technologies rely heavily on sophisticated tools and software to accurately capture the dentition. However, in order that these technologies are routinely used in a mainstream practice, a completely digital, highly accurate, and easily portable system needs to be established to create a worldwide information portal. A complete digital workflow will ensure that the appliances delivered are accurate and will be delivered efficiently to the consumer all over the world. Another more important benefit is that if appliances could be digitally built it would promise to reduce cost as the process would require less manual processing, and the transportation time and costs would not delay the fabrication process. It is this drive to create custom lab work that is fueling the next big game changer in orthodontics. The accurate representation of the dentition is by far the most important step to successful orthodontics. Traditional plaster casts are now slowly being replaced by digital models in orthodontics [1]. These digital models are often obtained via an indirect method that requires the transport of plaster casts or impressions of the dentition to a specialized company for laser or computer tomography (CT) scanning [2–5]. It is

a known fact that the process of making plaster casts from dental impression materials such as alginate and polyvinyl siloxane (PVS) impression material has always some degree of dimensional change. During transportation and the period between the impression procedure and the pouring of plaster in the impression, the dimensions of the impression and thus the accuracy of the plaster model can change. Impressions have to be sterilized, transported to a dental lab, and, after fabrication of the plaster models, transported again to the orthodontic office. Plaster dental models have then to be stored in the dental office and retrieved during orthodontic treatment and are prone to fracture. Plaster models and also dental impressions can be scanned with desktop scanners with laser beams and with dedicated CT scanners to transform these models and impressions into digital dental models (Figure 1.1).

In the literature it is reported that the accuracy of digital dental models scanned directly from impressions when compared to the "golden standard, the plaster cast" is sufficient for orthodontic analysis and treatment planning. But for this method to get a digital dental model an impression or a plaster model is required. As the impression taking procedure and the fabrication of plaster casts is an indirect method to get digital dental models, there is interest in the use of a direct method to copy the dentition.

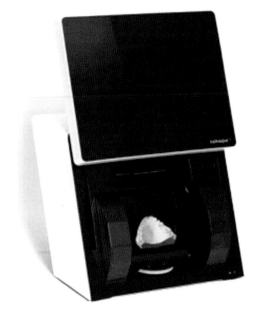

Figure 1.1 A dental model scanner.
Company: 3Shape.

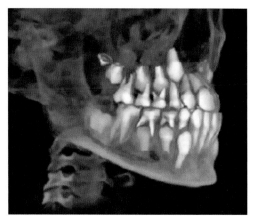

Figure 1.2 The segmented dentition on a CBCT radiograph.
Company: Anatomage Inc.

A direct method to capture the dentition is by using the cone beam computer tomography (CBCT) radiographs [6]. These radiographs can be used for dental analysis, but CBCT involves exposing the patient to radiation, and the quality of the dentition on the CBCT radiograph is directly related to the radiation dose used (Figure 1.2). Because of the ALARA principle (a radiation dose As Low As Reasonably Achievable), CBCT is not indicated for imaging of the dentition only.

To answer the need for a digital yet economical solution to physical impression materials, several companies have developed intraoral scanning systems to acquire digital intraoral impressions for any type of dental manufacturing. (For more information on the information presented in this chapter, please visit the websites of the companies mentioned.) Only intraoral scanning systems that can scan the entire dental arch can be used to replace orthodontic impression taking. The files of the scanners (stereolithographic (STL) files) can be used to produce digital dental models (Figure 1.3). These digital models can then be used with dedicated software for the diagnosis of a malocclusion, analyzing the dentition, digital treatment planning, and the design of dental, orthodontic, and surgical appliances. During the last decade, several intraoral scanners have been introduced. The first scanners introduced for

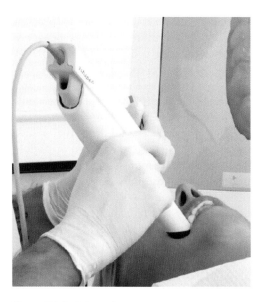

Figure 1.3 An intraoral scanner.
Company: 3Shape.

intraoral scanning had some disadvantages, such as the need for powdering the dentition, a slow scanning speed, and a relative large and heavy scanning head [7]. Intraoral scanners have recently come to the technology forefront in dentistry as the new holy grail, with the promise to eliminate the dreaded physical impression. If successfully adopted this is sure to be the next trend. Of course, at the end of the day, it will legitimately only be adopted if dentistry can be made easier, faster, and more precise.

It is easy with the intraoral scanners to scan the interarch relationship. Registration of the occlusion with an intraoral scanner does not require a separate material for bite registration. The occlusion can be quickly, directly, and accurately captured with the intraoral scanner (Figure 1.4). If intraoral scanners are used, the digital dental models are immediately available for diagnosis and analyzing a malocclusion.

Digital workflow using intraoral scanners

The images of the scanner (some scanners can be used to make a scan, color photographs, and an HD video taken at the same time) have the advantage that they can replace traditional plaster models (Figure 1.5) as well as photography of the dentition (Figure 1.6). Because intraoral scanning is a direct procedure, the intraoral scanning procedure could eventually become more accurate than traditional impression taking as intraoral scanning is not prone to some of

Figure 1.4 Scan of the occlusion. Company: 3Shape.

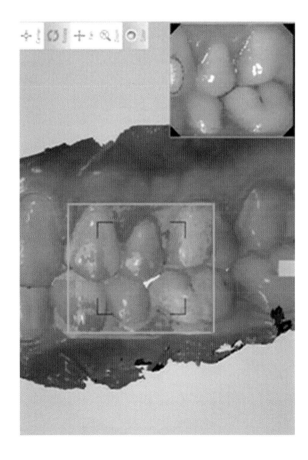

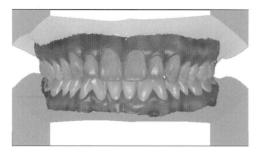

Figure 1.5 A digital dental model scanned with a color scanner.
Company: 3Shape.

the errors that can occur in the traditional impression taking procedure such as air bubbles, rupture of impression material, inaccurate impression tray dimensions, too much or too little impression material, inappropriate adhesion of the impression to the impression tray, and impression material distortion due to the disinfection and transportation procedure.

Inaccurate scanning can be improved by rescanning a specific part of the impression, so the procedure to entirely retake an impression can be postponed. Intraoral scanning could be particularly advantageous for patients with anxiety during impression taking (especially for the upper impression) and for cleft palate patients who could carry an increased risk of impression material aspiration and for whom standard impression

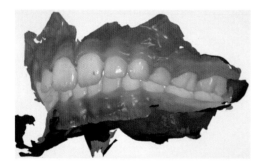

Figure 1.6 A intraoral scan in color.
Company: 3Shape.

trays are not suitable. Intraoral scanning could also be an advantage for patients currently undergoing orthodontic treatment with fixed appliances, for whom a traditional impression will be severely distorted because of the presence of the orthodontic appliances. Currently, the mean time needed for intraoral scanning is shorter than that required for taking traditional PVS impressions (one impression with heavy material and a second impression with soft impression material) but longer than required for the alginate impression taking procedure. Most patients have reported that the intraoral scanning procedure is more comfortable than conventional impression taking, especially with PVS impressions, although some studies have reported the opposite conclusion [8–11]. It can be speculated that the reduction in scanning time as well as the possibility to scan without powdering the dentition will improve the positive experience of the patient with the scanning procedure. It is expected that improvements of the scanners themselves will improve the speed, comfort, and accuracy of scanning. As an example, the advertisement of the recently introduced iTero intraoral scanner mentions a scanning time which is 20x faster compared to the older iTero intraoral scanner. Improvements in the scanning software further reduce the scanning time. A combination of a faster intraoral scanner and improved software and a faster computer (a computer with an Intel Core i7 processor and a fast NVIDIA video card and at least 16 GB of internal memory, can further reduce the scanning time. The technical procedure to scan the dentition, the alveolar bone, and the palate is not difficult. However, inexperienced practitioners will find completion of the first intraoral scans more time-consuming. Therefore, a practitioner's level of familiarity with the scanning system will substantially influence the time needed to complete the scans. Intraoral scanning of posterior teeth, especially third molars in patients with limited mouth opening, can sometimes be difficult. It can also be difficult to scan the bottom of the oral vestibule. This difficulty is related to the dimensions of the scanning tip and moisture control. The design of a thinner scanning tip may improve comfort during the scanning procedure.

Intraoral scanners generate stereolithographic (STL) files which are universally accepted for software programs and can be used to fabricate digital dental models for analysis and treatment planning. After treatment planning and the acceptance of the treatment plan by the patient, appliances should be selected and discussed with the patient.

These digital models, other digital documentation, and appliance designs can then be transferred to multiple industry platforms (digital labs) all over the world, and orthodontic appliances can be ordered regardless of brand. This new process of appliance manufacturing, known as the digital workflow, surely has the potential to affect all tenants of dentistry, not just orthodontics! For custom appliance fabrication, the quality of the digital impressions sent can be controlled by the dental lab, and after improvement of the digital impressions, production of the selected appliances can be started immediately. So the use of an intraoral scan reduces the time required to manufacture and deliver custom-made orthodontic appliances.

The cost of purchasing an intraoral scanner could be a profitable investment for an orthodontic office, as the intraoral scanning procedure will decrease the need to retake inaccurate dental impressions, as well as the need for impression disinfection and transportation. Additionally, the use of digital dental models will eliminate the need for dedicated space to store dental plaster casts in an orthodontic office. Another advantage is that the digital dental models are immediately available and can be used to discuss treatment with the patient during the documentation visit. It is important to get patients to believe in the quality and state of the art of the dental and orthodontic practice. Patients do understand if the office has invested in equipment that will make their experience of dental and orthodontic treatment better. Patients actually enjoy watching their scans build before their own eyes on screen. The intraoral scanner can be used as a marketing tool for the dental practice: if the patient agrees, the total scanning procedure can be displayed in the waiting room of the dental office and patients and their parents or other accompanying people can witness a life demonstration of the innovative procedures used in this specific dental office. After the completion of the scan, one of the dental staff members uploads the STL files and other digital patient files to the computers of a dental lab, or opens up the records on the computer software installed in their own dental office. Digital dental models can be easily shared with appliance manufacturers, colleagues, dental and medical specialists, and the patient.

Accuracy of digital dental models

Several studies evaluated the accuracy and reliability of digital dental models created with different acquisition methods, such as laser or light scanning of plaster casts, laser scanning of impressions, CT scanning of plaster casts and impressions, and intraoral scanning. These studies use different scanners and different software programs, which limits the ability to compare outcomes. Most of these studies found statistical differences in measurements on digital dental models compared to the same measurements made on dental plaster casts, but few of these measurement differences were clinically significant [6, 11–13].

Differences of more than 0.3 mm for the overjet, overbite, and tooth size (tooth diameter and tooth height), and of more than 0.4 mm for transverse and sagittal parameters, are generally considered clinically significant. For differences in the sum of six anterior teeth in the upper or lower dental arch, a threshold of 0.75 mm can be used. For the sum of 12 teeth in the upper or lower arch, a difference of 1.5 mm can be used to discriminate between statistically and clinically significant differences in measurements of dental models. Inadequate reference point localization may vary between examiners and will directly affect measurement reproducibility. Therefore, direct measurements on plaster casts or digital models are automatically associated with some degree of inaccuracy even when the points are precisely described. As the selected reference points for defining various measurements on plaster and digital dental models vary, the measuring method with calipers or computer software will not necessarily solve the problem of point identification, and so differences in measurements found cannot represent actual differences in measured distances. Point identification on digital models could be more accurate as the digital model can be enlarged and segmented for a better identification of the measuring points. Superimposition of digital dental models with dedicated software such as Geomagic and Maxillim is an alternative to compare the size and volume of the dentition and the alveolar bone on digital dental models. A color scale can then be used to evaluate differences in size and volume of digital dental models (Figure 1.7). Studies have shown that measurements made on plaster models may also not represent the actual dentition, because of possible dimensional changes in impression material and the process of fabricating the plaster cast. However, plaster casts have been used for analysis, treatment planning, and appliance fabrication for over 100 years. It has been reported by many dentists and orthodontists that the occlusion of the

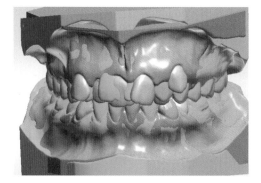

Figure 1.7 Superposition of two digital dental models.
Company: 3Shape.

digital models created by scanning a plaster cast or impression and the wax bite registration with a desktop scanner or a CT scanner can be inaccurate. If intraoral scanners are used, a direct method is used to register the relationship between the upper and lower dentition.

For some custom orthodontic appliances, impressions must be transported to other countries for planning and fabrication procedures. Alginate impression material is not sufficiently stable to be transported for more than a few days, so for fabrication of custom appliances in other countries PVS impressions or intraoral scans should be used as alternatives. The color images produced by this scanner will have a 1 : 1 ratio and could replace traditional intraoral imaging with photographs.

Conclusion

It can be expected that intraoral scanners will soon replace traditional impression taking procedures. The scanning time will decrease and the scanning head will become smaller. The intraoral scanning procedure is hygienic, images are immediately available, no transportation is needed, and storage and retrieval of the models is easy. The digital dental models can be easily shared with other people, enlarged, and clipped, and dedicated software is available for analyzing a case, planning treatment and appliance fabrication. The files of the scanner can be used in any dental lab. Furthermore, the intraoral color scans can replace traditional intraoral photographs and will have real colors and are presented in a 1 : 1 ratio.

References

1 Fleming, P.S., Marinho, V., and Johal, A. (2011) Orthodontic measurements on digital study models compared with plaster models: a systematic review. *Orthod. Craniofac. Res.*, **14**, 1–16.

2 Asquith, J., Gillgrass, T., and Mossey, P. (2007) Three-dimensional imaging of orthodontic models: a pilot study. *Eur. J. Orthod.*, **29**, 517–522.

3 Mullen, S.R., Martin, C.A., Ngan, P., and Gladwin, M. (2007) Accuracy of space analysis with emodels and plaster models. *Am. J. Orthod. Dentofacial Orthop.*, **132**, 346–352.

4 Stevens, D.R., Flores-Mir, C., Nebbe, B., *et al.* (2006) Validity, reliability, and reproducibility of plaster vs digital study models: comparison of peer assessment rating and Bolton analysis and their constituent measurements. *Am. J. Orthod. Dentofacial Orthop.*, **129**, 794–803.

5 Kusnoto, B. and Evans, C.A. (2002) Reliability of a 3D surface laser scanner for orthodontic applications. *Am. J. Orthod. Dentofacial Orthop.*, **122**, 342–348.

6 Wiranto, M.G., Engelbrecht, W.P., Tutein Nolthenius, H.E., *et al.* (2013) Validity, reliability, and reproducibility of linear measurements on digital models obtained from intraoral and cone-beam computed tomography scans of alginate impressions. *Am. J. Orthod. Dentofacial Orthop.*, **143**, 140–147.

7 Kravitz, N.D., Groth, C., Jones, P.E., *et al.* (2014) Intraoral digital scanners. *J. Clin. Orthod.*, **48**, 337–347.

8 Garino, F. and Garino, B. (2011) The OrthoCAD iOC intraoral scanner: a six-month user report. *J. Clin. Orthod.*, **45**, 161–164.

9 Vasudavan, S., Sullivan, S.R., and Sonis, A.L. (2010) Comparison of intraoral 3D scanning and conventional impressions for fabrication of orthodontic retainers. *J. Clin. Orthod.*, **44**, 495–497.

10 Yuzbasioglu, E., Kurt, H., Turunc, R., and Bilir, H. (2014) Comparison of digital and conventional impression techniques: evaluation of patients' perception, treatment comfort, effectiveness and clinical outcomes. *BMC Oral Health*, **14**, 10.

11 Grünheid, T., McCarthy, S.D., and Larson, B.E. (2014) Clinical use of a direct chairside oral scanner: an assessment of accuracy, time, and patient acceptance. *Am. J. Orthod. Dentofacial Orthop.*, **146**, 673–682.

12 Naidu, D. and Freer, T.J. (2013) Validity, reliability, and reproducibility of the iOC intraoral scanner: a comparison of tooth widths and Bolton ratios. *Am. J. Orthod. Dentofacial Orthop.*, **144**, 304–310.

13 Flügge, T.V., Schlager, S., Nelson, K., *et al.* (2013) Precision of intraoral digital dental impressions with iTero and extraoral digitization with the iTero and a model scanner. *Am. J. Orthod. Dentofacial Orthop.*, **144**, 471–478.

2

Documentation of the Face
K. Hero Breuning

Introduction

Cone beam computer tomography (CBCT) machines have entered the dental market. They can be used to make a range of three-dimensional (3D) images with different fields of view (FOVs) of the head in a 1 : 1 ratio. Simultaneously, some of these machines are capable of also making traditional two-dimensional (2D) radiographic images and a 3D facial scan to add texture to the radiographic image. By superimposition of the digital dental model, the CBCT, and the facial scan of a patient, a "virtual head" of that patient is available for diagnosis, treatment planning, and computer-aided design (CAD) and computer-aided manufacturing (CAM) procedures (Figure 2.1). Specific software (such as Anatomage, Dolphin, and 3Shape) can be used for diagnosis and treatment planning. This documentation of the face can also be used to plan maxillofacial surgery before or during orthodontic treatment [1–4].

Imaging of the skull in 3D

The usual 2D radiographs, such as lateral radiographics, have been used for orthodontic diagnosis and evaluation for many decades; the orthodontist B.H. Broadbent introduced the possible use of a lateral head plate for orthodontic treatment in 1931. In 1948, the first publication of an ortho pan tomographic (OPT) radiographic image was published. These 2D images have served very well during the past decades [5]. The head plate is mainly used to analyze the position of the maxilla, mandible, and the dentition in the skull. As some standard values for these data are available, the measurements of a specific patient can be compared with these standardized values. The head plate is not indicated to reveal medical problems: over-projection of structures and magnification of these images will limit the use of these images for diagnosis, treatment planning, and treatment evaluation in dentistry. Alan McLeod Cormack and Godfried Hounsfield introduced computed tomography (CT) radiographic images, which can be used for 3D evaluation of the skull in a 1 : 1 ratio, and thus expand the role of imaging. CT radiographic images can be used for diagnosis and for orthodontic and surgical treatment planning with dedicated third-party software. Some dentists will argue that these radiographs are expensive and need a relatively high radiation dose for imaging the skull. However, the development of CBCT machines which use a reduced amount of radiation will allow the orthodontist and maxillofacial surgeon to use 3D radiographs of the head as alternatives to traditional CT images.

Digital Planning and Custom Orthodontic Treatment, First Edition. Edited by K. Hero Breuning and Chung H. Kau.
© 2017 John Wiley & Sons, Inc. Published 2017 by John Wiley & Sons, Inc.

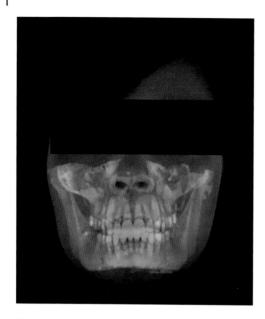

Figure 2.1 Superimposition of a facial scan, an intraoral scan, and a CBCT.
Company: Planmeca Oy.

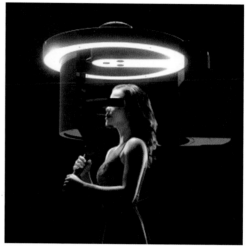

Figure 2.2 A 2D, 3D radiographic machine which can also make a facial scan.
Company: 3Shape.

The CBCT machines have been developed to make CT images of the skull. The radiographic head of the CBCT machine turns a full or a half circle around the head and a flat panel detector captures the photons and sends a signal to the computer. During the procedure, the patient stands or sits on a chair (Figure 2.2). Compared to the radiation dose needed for a CT scan, the radiation dose for these CBCTs of the head can be reduced. Furthermore, recent CBCT machines make a half turn around the head and, with the information collected, the computer is able to reconstruct a full head scan (of reduced quality). The newest CBCT machines can be used with "unlimited" selection possibilities of the FOV (the part of the skull which should receive a radiation dose). This FOV can be adjusted to the specific needs of each patient. The use of a dry run (a rotation of the device without radiation) to test the correct positioning of the patient and a "scout view" (a run with a very limited radiation dose, to

evaluate the accuracy of the FOV chosen) will further improve the quality of the image. For each radiograph, an estimation of the information presented in the radiographic image, which is needed for diagnosis and treatment planning and the possible risk for the development of cancer caused by the radiation used, should be balanced. After exposure, a powerful computer will reconstruct the data captured on the flat panel detector into a 3D image of the skull. Specific software can then be used to review the images of the skull on three planes. Usually, the CBCT can be reviewed with advanced imaging software (or simple DICOM viewers) from any angle, including axial, sagittal, and coronal cross-sectional slices of the skull (Figure 2.3). The files of the CBCT (DICOM files) can be changed with specific analyzing software to make certain parts of the image more visible by selecting specific Hounsfield values. Some of the well-known CBCT reviewing software programs for patients for orthodontic and maxillofacial surgery are Anatomage and Dolphin (Figure 2.4) [6]. Because the radiation dose of the older CBCT devices

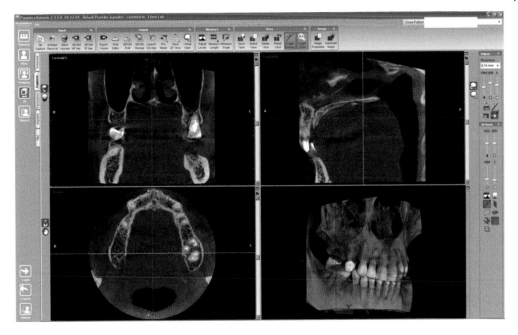

Figure 2.3 Slices of a CBCT used for evaluation.
Company: Planmeca Oy.

used for dentistry was higher compared to the dose needed for 2D radiographic images, specific indications for CBCT images were discussed and published in an attempt to agree on implement national and internationally accepted guidelines [7, 8]. However,

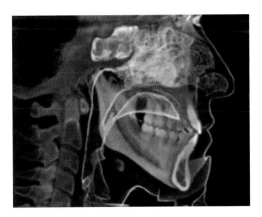

Figure 2.4 Segmentation of the airway in a CBCT.
Company: Dolphin Imaging & Management Solutions.

now that CBCT machines have been introduced recently that can make 3D radiographs with the same or even a reduced amount of radiation than that needed for making traditional OPT and head plate radiographs, these indications should be adjusted.

Careful selection of the FOV, the resolution of the images (voxel size), and the other settings to get the best image needed for diagnosis are still required.

CBCT machines have been recently developed to make different images, and CBCT imaging has become an essential component of the modern dental practices. When integrated with digital workflows, CBCT scans bring unparalleled insight to diagnostics and treatment procedures.

The Planmeca Oy ProMax machine was the first machine to combine three different types of 3D data capturing with one unit. This machine brings together the ability to make a CBCT image, a 3D facial photo (Figure 2.5) and a 3D dental model scan. The Planmeca

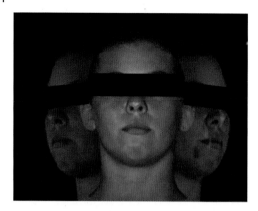

Figure 2.5 Facial photographs in 3D.
Company: Planmeca Oy.

Oy 4D Jaw Motion solution is able to track, record, and analyze jaw movement in 3D in real time. The same machine can also be used to make 2D radiographic images, including an OPT, without the need to change sensors. This machine is not indicated for making a 2D head plate of the skull. A disadvantage of this machine is the need to fix the head to prevent movement of the head during imaging. This fixing of the head gives rise to some distortion of the soft tissues of the face. The dedicated software for evaluation and to superimpose these images (Romexis software from Planmeca Oy) can be used to review, measure, and superimpose all the radiographic images but also the data from the 2D radiographs and the data captured with the intraoral scanner. After evaluation, the data can be stored in the Cloud and can be sent to colleagues, radiologists, medical specialists, the dental lab, and the patient. A free image viewer is available. For orthodontics, the software can be used for making a dental setup, and the design of some orthodontic appliances. An alternative CBCT machine capable of capturing radiographic 3D images of the skull, facial scans, a traditional OPT, and a traditional lateral head plate has been recently introduced: the 3Shape X1^{TM}. During scanning, the need for fixing the patient's head is not needed because of the use of a

tracking device on the head which monitors any movement of the head during the capturing procedure, which is then corrected during the reconstruction process. This machine combines CBCT, panoramic, cephalogram, and face scanning in one system. The low dose and rotating shutter technology should improve image quality and reduction of radiation dose. The use of the "dynamic field of view" enables adjustable FOV at the touch of a button. The software is capable of merging CBCT and panoramic scans with digital impressions and face scans to create a digital patient for diagnostics, treatment planning, and appliance fabrication. The integrated outputs for all images of this machine are in the standard DICOM format, so they can be exported to the software of choice. Of course, the 3Shape dental practice software solutions that merge CBCT and intraoral scans and the files of the intraoral scanner can be used for integrated diagnostics, planning, and appliance fabrication.

The CBCT images are used by the suresmile company during the planning and evaluation of orthodontic treatment (Figure 2.6). After segmentation of the dentition, it is possible to make a dental setup with the suresmile software. In this planning process the dental roots can be positioned in the alveolar bone. As the dental crowns from

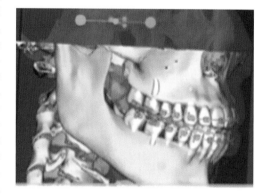

Figure 2.6 A CBCT with simulated movement of the mandible.
Company: suresmile.

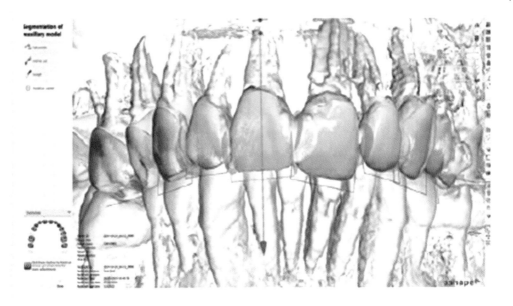

Figure 2.7 Superimposition of an intraoral scan and a CBCT.
Company: 3Shape.

an intraoral scan can be merged with the dentition on the CBCT, the need for follow-up CBCTs using specific software such as suresmile or 3Shape's Ortho-Analyser can be reduced (Figure 2.7). If an initial CBCT is available, a progress intraoral scan can be used to review the root position of a specific case. The quality of the scanned brackets as seen on CBCT radiographs is not accurate, so the scanned brackets and the image of the brackets on the CBCT can be merged. This process is needed to enable custom wire fabrication after approval of the setup by the orthodontist.

Discussion

In the past, several devices were needed to make 2D and 3D radiographic images, and for facial scanning a laser scanner or a series of cameras was used. As described in Chapter 1, digital dental models were made with CT scanners, laser scanners, or intraoral scanners. The introduction of machines capable of capturing both radiographic and facial images and the possibility to use integrated software to review these different images and intraoral scans was a big step forward. The software developed by several companies can now be used for analysis of the patient, treatment planning (including orthodontic, surgical and prosthetic treatment), and for the design and fabrication of dental restorations, prosthetic devices, dentures, temporomandibular joint (TMJ) splints, implant placement splints, surgical splints, and of course for the fabrication of orthodontic appliances. Storage of the data in the Cloud and easy communication with the dental lab, dental and medical colleagues, and the patient is a huge step toward the desired direction of a digital workflow. It can be expected that the quality of this "virtual head" for diagnosis, treatment planning, and treatment evaluation will continue to improve. The fourth dimension (movement) should be added to enable evaluation of the occlusion, the TMJ, and other functional movements of the face.

References

1 Plooij, J.M., Swennen, G.R., Rangel, F.A., *et al.* (2009) Evaluation of reproducibility and reliability of 3D soft tissue analysis using 3D stereophotogrammetry. *Int. J. Oral. Maxillofac. Surg.*, **38** (3), 267–73.

2 Maal, T.J., van Loon, B., Plooij, J.M., *et al.* (2010) Registration of 3-dimensional facial photographs for clinical use. *J. Oral. Maxillofac. Surg.*, **68** (10), 2391–2401.

3 Hodges, R.J., Atchison, K.A., White, S.C. (2013) Impact of cone-beam computed tomography on orthodontic diagnosis and treatment planning. *Am. J. Orthod. Dentofacial. Orthop.*,**143** (5), 665–674.

4 Liebregts, J.H., Timmermans, M., De Koning, M.J., *et al.* (2015) Three-dimensional facial simulation in bilateral sagittal split osteotomy: a validation study of 100 patients. *J. Oral. Maxillofac. Surg.*, **73** (5), 961–970.

5 Rischen, R.J., Breuning, K.H., Bronkhorst, E.M., and Kuijpers-Jagtman, A.M. (2013) Records needed for orthodontic diagnosis and treatment planning: a systematic review. *PLoS One*, **8** (11), e74186.

6 Paula, L.K., Solon-de-Mello, P. de A., Mattos, C.T., *et al.* (2015) Influence of magnification and superimposition of structures on cephalometric diagnosis. *Dental Press. J. Orthod.*, **20** (2), 29–34.

7 van Vlijmen, O.J., Kuijpers, M.A., Bergé, S.J., *et al.* (2012) Evidence supporting the use of cone-beam computed tomography in orthodontics. *J. Am. Dent. Assoc.*, **143** (3), 241–252.

8 Kuijpers-Jagtman, A.M., Kuijpers, M.A.R., Schols, J.G.J.H., *et al.* (2013) The use of cone-beam computed tomography for orthodontic purposes. *Seminars in Orthodontics*, **September**.

3

Dynamic Motion Capture of the Mandible
Shushu He and Chung H. Kau

Introduction

Temporomandibular joints (TMJ), together with the occlusion, the masticatory muscles, and the vascular and nervous systems supplying these tissues, constitute the stomatognathic system. The mandibular movement executed by TMJ is a motor functional movement that reflects the command of all these components and is critical not only for oral-related function such as food taking and speech but also for the systematic, mental, and physical functions of the body [1]. Jaw recording is thus important for the understanding of the normal function of the stomatognathic system and for the diagnosis and treatment of TMJ disorders and diseases.

Various devices have been developed to record and analyze the mandibular movement for more than a century [2]. There are methods using mechanical devices with graphical methods involving marking needles and recording styli and pantographs, and almost all these methods have the disadvantage of causing interference with jaw movements [3]. Photographic techniques require complicated manual transference to produce tracings of jaw movements, which can introduce erroneous measurements [2]. Roentgenographic methods with radiation exposure have been used in the past but may not be allowed by ethical review committees for experimental purposes nowadays.

Two systems of magnetometry, the mandibular kinesiograph, and the sirognathograph, which depend on the changes in the magnetic flux occurring when a small bar magnet moves relative to a sensor, have been used to measure mandibular movements in three dimensions for a long time. These devices are found not to interfere with the mandible movements. Opto-electronic tracking systems obtain mandibular movements by using cameras to tracking the spatial position of light-emitting diodes [4]. They also have an advantage of disturbing the individual's chewing pattern less than normal chewing function [5].

These methods alone, however, didn't include the TMJ joints and their nearby anatomy structures into measurements. Three-dimensional (3D) TMJ joint morphology has been reconstructed by spiral and helical computed tomography (CT) and magnetic resonance imaging (MRI). Data have been merged with jaw movement recordings by ultrafast MRI, electromagnetic tracking device, or opto-electric measuring systems in a few previous studies [4, 6]. The disadvantage of MRI imaging is that the patient must lie down on the scan bed, which might alter the mandibular movement. Also, MRI imaging of bony anatomy is never visually clear. One of the main disadvantages of CT imaging comes from radiation exposure. Also the visualization of patient-specific jaw

Digital Planning and Custom Orthodontic Treatment, First Edition. Edited by K. Hero Breuning and Chung H. Kau.
© 2017 John Wiley & Sons, Inc. Published 2017 by John Wiley & Sons, Inc.

movement and chewing pattern has not been clearly presented before.

At present, there are dynamic systems to understand the TMJ. The SiCAT Function (SiCAT, Bonn, Germany) can directly combine and merge 3D cone beam computed tomography (CBCT) and electronic jaw motion tracking (JMT) data. CBCT, which offers a 3D image of facial and dental structures, has been widely used in the dental field [7]. The SiCAT JMT system is an electronic recording system that is based on 3D ultrasound measurements. The ultrasound-based system converts the propagation times of multiple acoustic signals into spatial information, which therefore could record the lower jaw movements of the patient in all degrees of freedom.

JMT system

At present, the JMT system is a closed one. All data acquired must be obtained through the Sirona or SiCAT Platform. This provides the advantage that the system is seamless and transitions from one stage to the other easily. The disadvantage is that the hardware needs to be purchase solely for this purpose.

CBCT

As a routine treatment record, a CBCT is taken for a patient. As a preparation, silicone impression material is put in both the maxillary and mandibular side of the FusionBite reference tray and the patient is normally asked to bite on the impression material (Figure 3.1a). During CBCT scanning, the patient wears the FusionBite reference tray with the silicone impression in their mouth. There are eight radiopaque markers on the FusionBite tray, which will serve as landmarks for the fusion of CBCT data and JMT data. The CBCT device (Sirona Galileos, Bensheim, Germany) is used, which acquires the images

with a scan time of 14s, capture the maxilla-mandibular region in a 210° rotation, and has a reported radiation dosage of only 29 μSi to 54 μSi according to the manufacturer. The field of view is a spherical volume of 15 cm. The voxel size is between 0.15 mm and 0.30 mm and the grayscale is 12 bit. The acquired CBCT data were transferred from the scanner to a workstation, where 3D images were constructed by GALAXIS 3D software (Sirona Galileos, Bensheim, Germany). The data are saved as DICOM (digital imaging and communication in medicine) format.

Preparation of the jaw tracking system

The para-occlusal T-attachment is contoured according to the low jaw dental arch. Auto-polymerizing composite is applied to the bent part of the T-attachment, and adapted to the tooth surfaces or to the study model. A short setting time for the material is required (Figure 3.1b). Remove excess material and sharp edges and make sure the upper teeth are not in touch with the attachment in order to guarantee an undisturbed functional movement of the jaw in the occlusion.

Tracking system

The upper jaw sensor is positioned stably on the patient's head. It is important to ensure that the upper headband is on the patient's skull and that the nose pads don't stretch the skin in the nasion area. The elastic rear headband is tightened comfortably for the patient. Place the SiCAT FusionBite tray (previously adapted with silicone impression) into the mouth and make sure the patient bites into the right position. In some instances, medical glue might be needed to secure the T-attachment firmly in the patient's mouth. Once this is done, the SiCAT JMT$^+$ software

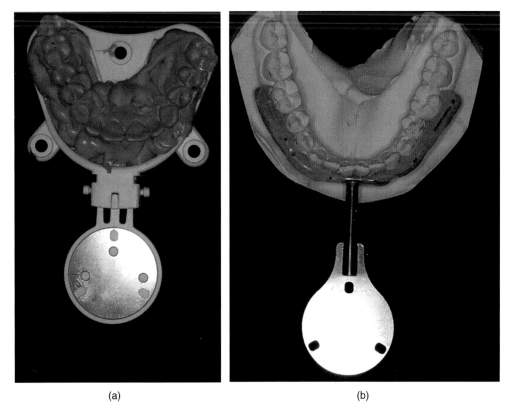

(a)   (b)

Figure 3.1 Preparation of jaw moving tracking; (a) FusionBite reference tray with impression material; (b) adapt T-attachment with auto-polymerizing composite to study model.
Company: Sirona Dental Systems, Inc.

is employed. The following steps should be performed next:

- Attach the SiCAT JMT$^+$ lower jaw sensor to the SiCAT FusionBite.
- Click "record" and the software will guide the program throughout the calibration sequence.
- Remember to always keep the SiCAT FusionBite in the mouth and attach the lower jaw sensor to the para-occlusal T-attachment, and then press "record."
- Take out the SiCAT FusionBite. The functional jaw movement such as opening, right, and left lateral movement, protrusive, and chewing can be recorded.

Data fusion

Once the above has been completed, load the CBCT data and JMT files in the software SiCAT Function suite. Choose any three radiopaque markers on the FusionBite tray (Figure 3.2a) and the tray will be automatically located, as in Figure 3.2b, and the CBCT and JMT data can be merged automatically.

Segmentation of the mandible

Segmentation of the mandible can be performed semi-automatically in the software. When the approximate position of the mandible is indicated by drawing marks on

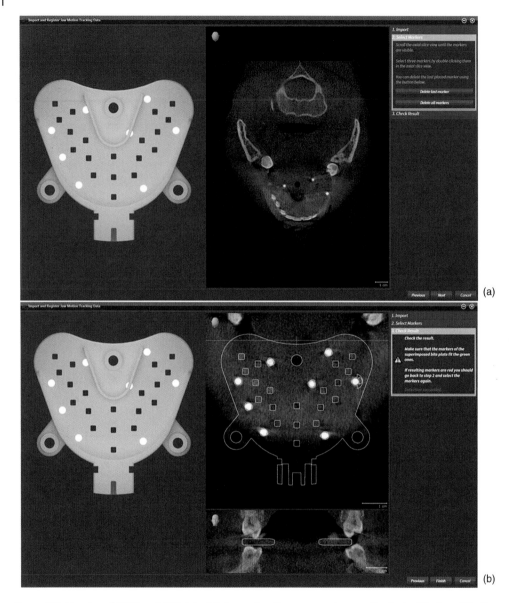

Figure 3.2 Merging of CBCT and JMT data; (a) choose 3 radiopaque markers on the FusionBite tray; (b) other radiopaque markers were found and the tray was located.
Company: Sirona Dental Systems, Inc.

the radiographic sectional slices, the software will calculate the data and present a 3D image of the cropped mandibular segment on the screen (Figure 3.3). The blue color is used to represent the mandible and the green color for the fossa.

Recording of mandibular movement by SiCAT JMT$^+$

Mandibular movements—including opening, right/left lateralization, and protrusive—can be recorded and re-recorded at any

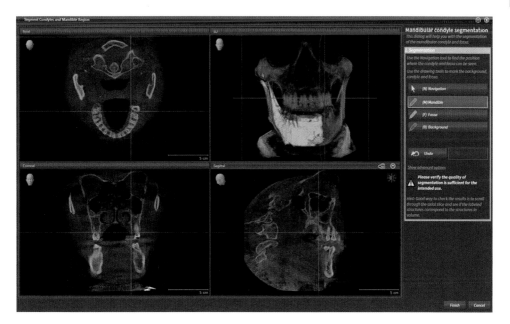

Figure 3.3 Segmentation of the mandible.
Company: Sirona Dental Systems, Inc.

time. The ranges of these movements are automatically displayed and correspond well to the patient's movement.

Merge of CBCT and JMT data in SiCAT suite

Once the mandible DICOM is successfully segmented, merging of CBCT and JMT data can occur. The visualization of patient-specific movement of the mandible, including the condyles, is displayed and is now an exact replica of the patient's mandibular movement. In the dynamic mode, the movement path of any selected point of the condyle and the mandible body such as inter-incisal point movement of the lower mandibular teeth is depicted on the trace. Selected tracing images of the movement are presented in Figures 3.4, 3.5, and 3.6. Based on the anatomical information provided by the CBCT data, we could not only see the movement of the mandible but also see the movement of the condyle in the patient's fossa.

Discussion

Traditional recording of the condylar movements

Jaw tracking devices and methods in the past have greatly improved the understanding of mandibular movements. However, easier and better devices and methods are still needed for the accurate evaluation and extensive exploration of the normal and diseased functions of TMJ joints. This chapter shows that the SiCAT Function software relates JMT data with individual imaging data and provides visualization of true condylar movements.

The ranges of all the movements are easily obtained immediately after the recording, and from the tracing images the routes of the movements are clearly presented. In a previous study, the recordings on three sequential days showed that this method has high repeatability. The data, however, were not exactly the same and therefore can vary from patient to patient.

Opening

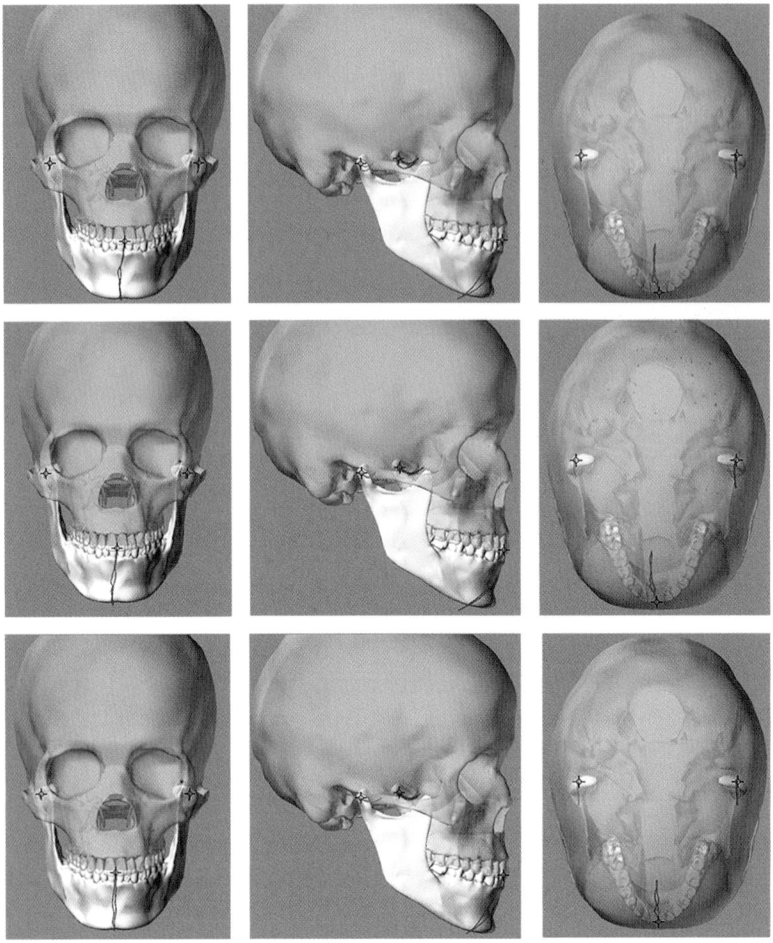

(a)

Figure 3.4 Tracing images in selected planes by JMT during (a) opening; (b) right lateral movement; (c) left lateral movement; and (d) protrusion.
Company: Sirona Dental Systems, Inc.

Future directions

The SiCAT Function software provides measurement and visualization of mandibular movement. Also, it provides a way to predict the position of the condyle without extra radioactive exposure when the tooth is in specific occlusion. Further studies can verify the repeatability of the SiCAT Function software and orthodontists could use the system to study the movement of healthy and diseased TMJ joints, to diagnose patients with jaw deformities, and to help treat TMJ problems.

Conclusion

The SiCAT Function software is a system capable of measuring and visualizing patient-specific jaw movement relative to the patient-specific anatomy of the jaw.

Lateral right

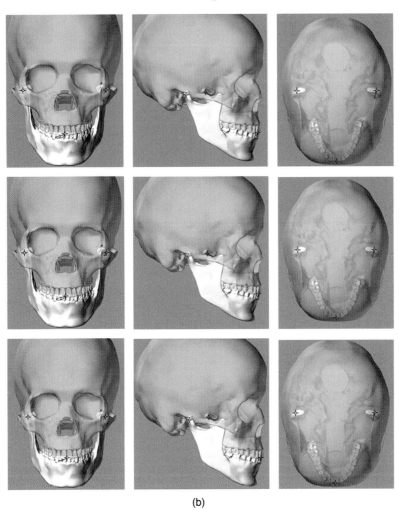

(b)

Figure 3.4 (*Continued*)

Lateral left

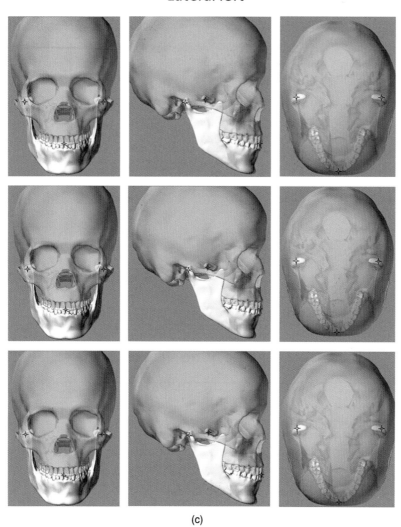

(c)

Figure 3.4 (*Continued*)

Protrusion

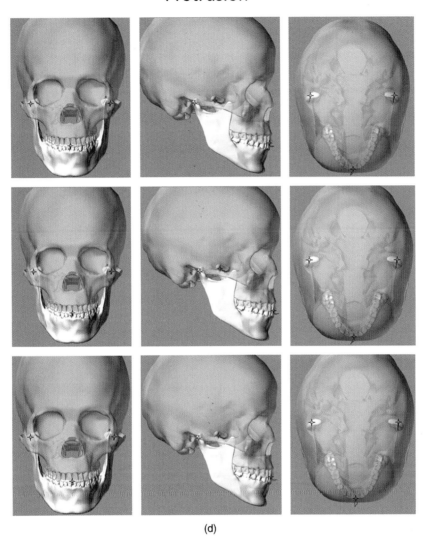

(d)

Figure 3.4 (*Continued*)

Opening (condyle)

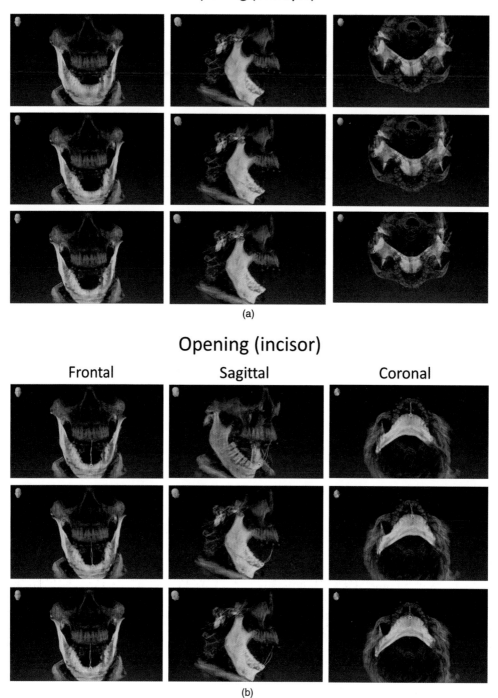

(a)

Opening (incisor)

| Frontal | Sagittal | Coronal |

(b)

Figure 3.5 Patient-specific visualization of mandibular opening movement: (a) condyle pathway; (b) incisor pathway.
Company: Sirona Dental Systems, Inc.

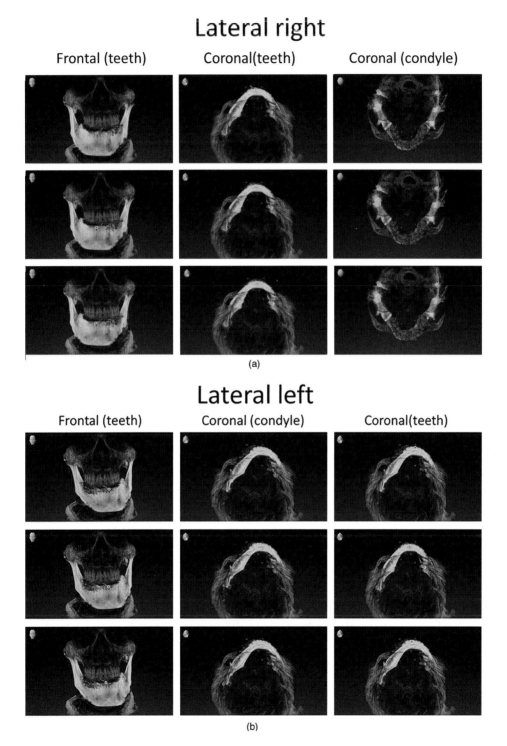

Lateral right

Frontal (teeth) Coronal(teeth) Coronal (condyle)

(a)

Lateral left

Frontal (teeth) Coronal (condyle) Coronal(teeth)

(b)

Figure 3.6 Patient-specific visualization of mandibular lateral movement: (a) lateral right; (b) lateral left. Company: Sirona Dental Systems, Inc.

References

1 Nakata, M. (1998) Masticatory function and its effects on general health. *Int. Dent. J.*, **48**, 540–548.

2 Howell, P.G., Johnson, C.W., Ellis, S., *et al.* (1992) The recording and analysis of EMG and jaw tracking: I: the recording procedure. *J. Oral Rehabil.*, **19**, 595–605.

3 Soboleva, U., Laurina, L., and Slaidina, A. (2005) Jaw tracking devices: historical review of methods development: part I. *Stomatologija*, 7, 67–71.

4 Terajima, M., Endo, M., Aoki, Y., *et al.* (2008) Four-dimensional analysis of stomatognathic function. *Am. J. Orthod. Dentofacial Orthop.*, **134**, 276–287.

5 Soboleva, U., Laurina, L., and Slaidina, A. (2005) Jaw tracking devices: historical review of methods development: part II. *Stomatologija*, 7, 72–76.

6 Baltali, E., Zhao, K.D., Koff, M.F., *et al.* (2008) A method for quantifying condylar motion in patients with osteoarthritis using an electromagnetic tracking device and computed tomography imaging. *J. Oral Maxillofac. Surg.*, **66**, 848–857.

7 Liu, D.G., Zhang, W.L., Zhang, Z.Y., *et al.* (2008) Localization of impacted maxillary canines and observation of adjacent incisor resorption with cone-beam computed tomography. *Oral Surg. Oral. Med. Oral Pathol. Oral Radiol. Endod.*, **105**, 91–98.

4

Analysis of Digital Dental Documentation

K. Hero Breuning and Chung H. Kau

Introduction

Because dentists and dental specialists are used to using plaster dental models with a specific design, the raw stereolithographic (STL) files of the scanned dentition should be used to make digital "study models" which should look like the familiar plaster models used in "the old days." This digital model fabrication process can be performed in a dental lab or in the dental or orthodontic office [1, 2]. A wireless Internet connection in the office or at home can be used for easy access transfer and efficient communication between the dentist, the dental office, the dental lab, and the providers of custom orthodontic appliances [3].

The dentist, orthodontist, maxillofacial surgeon, and lab technician will be able to discuss and share cases, review treatment proposals, and simulate treatment plans online (Figure 4.1).

For the analysis of the dental and skeletal problems, the intraoral scan, the two-dimensional (2D) or three-dimensional (3D) radiograph, and the 3D facial scan should be efficiently and accurate merged by the analyzing software [4, 5]. Dedicated software programs should be used to analyze the digital dental model, the 2D and 3D radiographs, and the facial scan in a systematic and effective standardized process (Figure 4.2).

In recent software programs, such as 3Shape's Ortho-Analyser, all traditional methods to analyze digital dental models—such as the analysis of tooth dimension, distances between teeth, the Bolton ratio, space requirements, dental arc shapes, and the traditional measuring of the overjet and overbite—will be recorded semi-automatically [6]. During this process, it can be helpful to magnify and use clipping procedures to increase the accuracy of the measuring and analyzing procedures (Figure 4.3). Because the digital dental models can be merged with the cone beam computer tomography (CBCT) radiographs and the facial scan, the position of the teeth (extremely helpful for cases with impacted or supernumerary teeth) can be accurately reviewed [7]. In a "virtual head," dental, facial, and skeletal analysis should be performed and recorded in a systematic way. Of course, this extensive analysis takes time, but because all the data are available in an integrated digital file, the quality of the analysis

Digital Planning and Custom Orthodontic Treatment, First Edition. Edited by K. Hero Breuning and Chung H. Kau.
© 2017 John Wiley & Sons, Inc. Published 2017 by John Wiley & Sons, Inc.

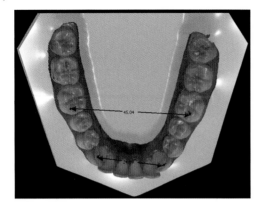

Figure 4.1 Measurements on a digital dental model. Company: 3Shape.

can be optimized. Software programs such as Anatomage and Dolphin can be used to visualize specific parts of the CBCT radiograph such as the airway, the bone, or the dentition [8, 9]. The facial scan can be used for evaluation of the profile, the symmetry of the face, and so on. If possible, not only static images should be analyzed. In some software programs (such as Ortho-Analyser), the occlusion can be reviewed with different virtual articulators (Figure 4.4). Some software programs (suresmile by OraMetrix and Romexis software by Planmeca) enable practitioners to simulate the movement of the mandible on CBCT images. (For more information on the topics mentioned in this chapter, please visit the websites of the companies mentioned.) A static facial scan can be made by some "all in one" CBCT machines or with a specific facial scanner (3dMD or facial laser scanners) (Figure 4.5). A dynamic facial scan (four-dimensional images), including recording of the speech, is possible with systems such as the 3dMD Face and 3dMD Trio systems [10].

After analyzing the documentation, a total report of this analysis, including some relevant images, should be made and sent to the referring dentist and other healthcare professionals. Most data needed for making this report are provided by the software.

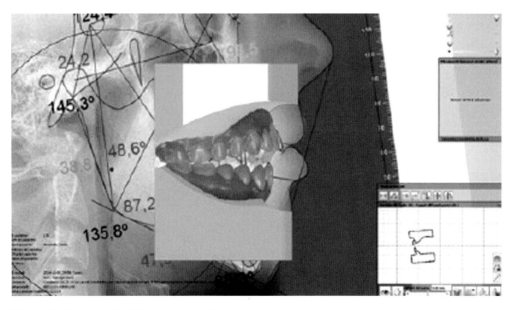

Figure 4.2 Matching of a digital dental model and a cephalogram. Company: 3Shape.

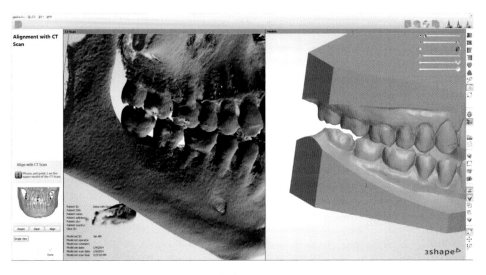

Figure 4.3 A CBCT and a digital dental model before superimposition.
Company: 3Shape.

Figure 4.4 A virtual articulator for digital dental models.
Company: 3Shape.

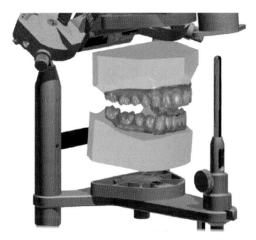

Figure 4.5 A machine for capturing facial scans, facial motion, and sound.
Company: 3dMD.

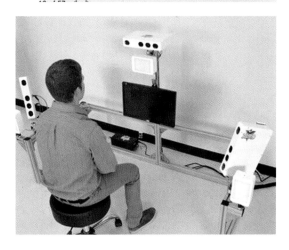

References

1 Rossini, G., Parrini, S., Castroflorio, T., *et al.* (2016) Diagnostic accuracy and measurement sensitivity of digital models for orthodontic purposes: a systematic review. *Am. J. Orthod. Dentofacial Orthop.*, **149**, 161–170.

2 Martin, C.B., Chalmers, E.V., Mclntyre, G.T., *et al.* (2015) Orthodontic scanners: what's available?, *J. Orthod.*, **42** (2), 136–143.

3 Zimmermann, M. and Mehl, A. (2015) Virtual smile design systems: a current review. *Int. J. Comput. Dent.*, **18**, 303–317.

4 Joda, T., Brägger, U., and Gallucci, G. (2015) Systematic literature review of digital three-dimensional superimposition techniques to create virtual dental patients. *Int. J. Oral. Maxillofac. Implants*, **30**, 330–337.

5 Joda, T. and Gallucci, G.O. (2015) The virtual patient in dental medicine. *Clin. Oral Implants Res.*, **26** (6), 725–726.

6 Czarnota, J., Hey, J., and Fuhrmann, R. (2016) Measurements using orthodontic analysis software on digital models obtained by 3D scans of plaster casts: intrarater reliability and validity. *J. Orofac. Orthop.* **77** (1), 22–30.

7 Ghoneima, A., Allam, E., Kula, K., and Windsor, L.J. (2012) Three-dimensional imaging and software advances in orthodontics, in *Orthodontics: Basic aspects and clinical considerations* (ed. F. Bourzgui), InTech, Rijeka, Croatia.

8 Weissheimer, A., Menezes, L.M., Sameshima, G.T., *et al.* (2012) Imaging software accuracy for 3-dimensional analysis of the upper airway. *Am. J. Orthod. Dentofacial Orthop.*, **142**, 801–813.

9 El, H. and Palomo, J.M. (2010) Measuring the airway in 3 dimensions: a reliability and accuracy study. *Am. J. Orthod. Dentofacial Orthop.*, **137**, S50, e51–59, discussion S50–52.

10 Tzou, C.H., Artner, N.M., Pona, I., *et al.* (2014) Comparison of three-dimensional surface-imaging systems. *J. Plast. Reconstr. Aesthet. Surg.*, **67**, 489–497.

5

Orthodontic Treatment Planning

K. Hero Breuning and Chung H. Kau

Introduction

Once a case has been analyzed, the process of treatment planning can begin. The segmented dental crowns and, if available, the segmented dentition on the cone beam computer tomography (CBCT) radiographs can now be used to simulate the dental movement needed to correct a malocclusion using virtual repositioning software (Figure 5.1). A setup of the dentition can then be made (Figure 5.2) [1–4]. Depending on the preference of the dentist, orthodontist, or maxillofacial surgeon, this process can be done by a dental technician or by the orthodontist with dedicated software. If the initial setup is outsourced to a dental lab technician, uploading of the digital documentation of the patient to the computers of the lab is required. Some orthodontic labs use a file transfer protocol (FTP) to enable the easy and safe uploading of the files. These FTP servers are built on a client server architecture and use separate control and data connections between the client and the server. FTP users may authenticate themselves using a "clear-text sign-in" protocol, normally in the form of a username and password, but can connect anonymously if the server is configured to allow it. Secure transmission protects the username and password, and encrypts the content.

The setup

Traditionally, the dental crowns (segmented teeth of the plaster models) were positioned with dental wax into an ideal position. This method was introduced by Harold Kesling in 1953 and this was then used to fabricate a "positioner": a flexible orthodontic finishing appliance made on the setup, which could be used to finish orthodontic treatment (Figure 5.3).

Kesling later detected the value of this setup for the planning of orthodontic treatment. A dental setup has now been recognized as a valuable diagnostic tool for orthodontic, dental, and surgical treatment, which can be used to confirm, modify, or reject a planned treatment plan. The original technique to make a setup has been improved over time as it was understood that there should be a reference for making a setup. One of the references used for the traditional setup in plaster and wax is the position of the lower incisor as displayed on the cephalometric radiograph. The procedure to make a traditional setup is then started with the positioning of the lower incisors. After positioning the lower incisors, wax or resin stops are placed in the posterior region of the model to maintain the vertical dimension of the dentition after removal of the crowns of teeth from the plaster model. An alternative

Digital Planning and Custom Orthodontic Treatment, First Edition. Edited by K. Hero Breuning and Chung H. Kau.
© 2017 John Wiley & Sons, Inc. Published 2017 by John Wiley & Sons, Inc.

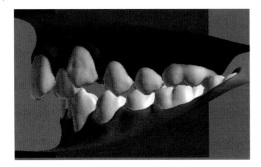

Figure 5.1 Segmented crowns of a digital model. Company: Exceed-Ortho.

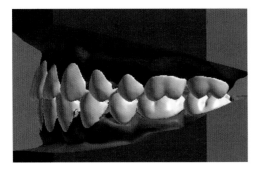

Figure 5.2 Setup of the segmented crowns. Company: Exceed-Ortho.

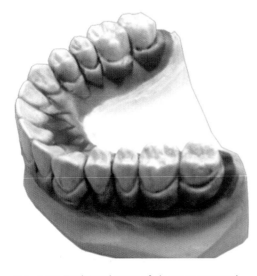

Figure 5.3 Traditional setup of plaster crowns and wax.
Company: Picture by Dr. Breuning.

way to maintain the horizontal position of the teeth is to retain the last molars in the plaster model and use them as vertical references. A disadvantage of using a plaster model for a dental setup is that the plaster model should first be copied and, second, the setup procedure is quite time-consuming. The superimposition of these traditional setups and initial plaster models is not possible [5].

As software programs are now available to make a virtual setup for digital dental models much faster, without the need for physical dental models, this virtual treatment planning should be used not only for difficult cases but also for cases which should be treated with a multidisciplinary approach (Figure 5.4) [6]. A virtual setup can now be considered a standard procedure for the planning of each orthodontic treatment. For making a digital setup, the dental crowns should be segmented from the digital dental model, using software, for instance the Insignia software, for virtual segmentation (Figure 5.4). After segmentation, a reference for the dentition based on the original dentition and the alveolar bone should be selected (Figure 5.5). In some setup software programs, such as Ortho-Analyser, the occlusal plane and the palatal midline are defined as reference planes. Then an automatic suggestion for segmentation will be presented by the software. This segmentation process is done in most software programs in a semi-automatic way. Manual improvement of the suggested segmentation line by the dentist or technician is needed (Figure 5.6), especially when a dentition with braces has been scanned. The axis and direction of the root should then be indicated on the dental crowns, before the actual segmentation procedure can be started. After segmentation, virtual roots ("avatars") will be added to the dental crowns according to the planned direction of the roots. The estimated rotation point of each tooth, as suggested by the software, should be corrected before the actual segmentation.

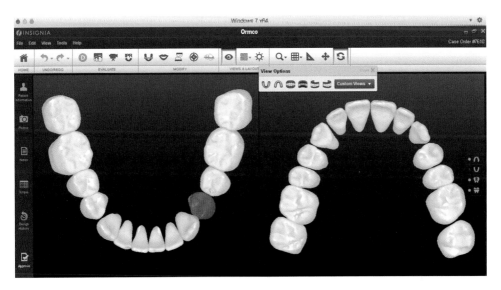

Figure 5.4 A setup can be used for multidisciplinary treatment planning.
Company: Ormco.

The next step in an analyzing program such as Ortho-Analyser is the actual segmentation which will be done automatically according to the segmentation lines on the digital model. After this segmentation, the "sculpture" function can be used to remove some small failures in the digital impression of dental crowns. The position of the dental crowns can now be changed with the software to make a setup of the planned treatment. During the making of a setup, the available space in the alveolar arch can be evaluated by reviewing the alveolar bone as displayed on the digital model. In some

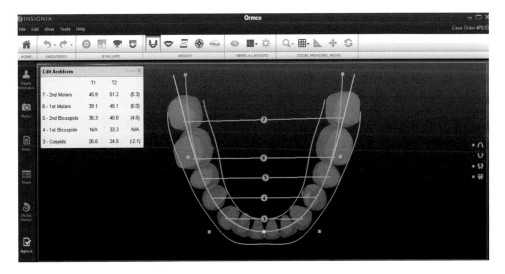

Figure 5.5 Outline of the alveolar bone for setup fabrication.
Company: Ormco.

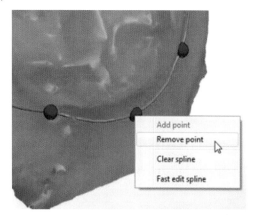

Add point
Remove point
Clear spline
Fast edit spline

Figure 5.6 Segmentation line for dental crowns. Company: 3Shape.

software programs, such as Ortho-Analyser, a virtual arch wire can be designed for the mandibular and maxillary dentition on the original digital dental model. These arches can then be used as a reference during the process of making the setup. The "smile line" should be evaluated when the patient is in the orthodontic office for consultation and should be captured on photographs, the facial scan, a video, and, if indicated, on the CBCT. If a CBCT is available, the digital scan of the dental crowns can be superimposed (merged) on the crowns of the dentition on the CBCT. Information from several sources for three-dimensional imaging of the skull (a "virtual head") allows evaluation of the available alveolar bone and can be used to estimate the effect of the planned tooth (and jaw) movement on the soft tissues.

CBCT images are used by companies, such as suresmile, during their planning and evaluation of orthodontic treatment. With the suresmile software, it is also possible to make a dental setup after segmentation of the dentition.

A major advantage of the use of a CBCT for planning of orthodontic treatment is the possibility to evaluate and correct the position of the roots in relation to the alveolar bone in treatment planning. Ideally, these

simulations will also show the possible therapeutic outcome of the orthodontic treatment of the dentition and the changes in the soft tissues that can be expected. This virtual treatment plan will also reveal the need for tooth extraction or interproximal stripping, depending on the malocclusion of the individual patient and their esthetic wishes. These CBCT images can be used during setup manufacturing to correct or improve the smile line in the setup.

In the software, values which limit the maximum amount of tooth movement can be selected, so application of excessive tooth movement in the setup in relation to the reference planes will not be possible. Grids can be used to control the symmetry of the setup. Clipping functions can be used to evaluate relations between the teeth and between the arches (including contact points and occlusal stops). One single tooth or a group of teeth can be moved at the same time during making the setup. Occlusal contacts should be evaluated and corrected in the setup when needed (Figure 5.7). A color scale can be used to show the contact points in the setup. The original digital dental model and the setup can be evaluated in a virtual articulator, to evaluate the actual and planned functional contacts and occlusion. During this process of virtually moving teeth, the dentist or technician is able to quantify and visualize the applied tooth movement. Obviously, tooth movement has its biological limitations. Too much expansion or compression of the dental arches may result in unstable results and periodontal recessions. So, the setup should be made based on biological principles and clinical experience. The role of the orthodontist during this setup fabrication is very important, because the technician will not be able to decide about the need for expansion of the dental arches or interdental reduction of tooth material ("stripping"), or whether to extract teeth. If a lab technician makes the setup, a treatment plan should be available and after making the

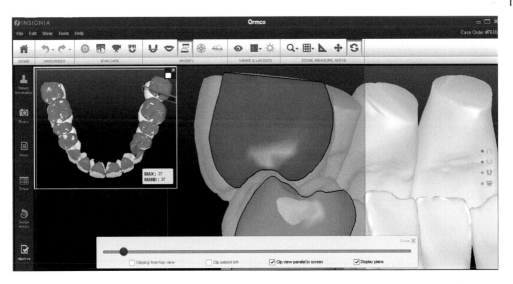

Figure 5.7 Occlusion planning for a setup.
Company: Ormco.

setup the planned virtual treatment should be sent to the orthodontist for evaluation. The original tooth position and changes in dental position introduced in the setup should be recorded and available for further reference.

Example of digital planning for a custom buccal brace (Insignia) system

The workflow for a custom appliance system for buccal brackets, called Insignia, starts with documentation in the orthodontic office. The orthodontist sends a set of polyvinyl siloxane (PVS) impressions with bite registration or an intraoral scan to the company. The orthodontist has to fill in an ordering sheet online on the secured website of the company for each new patient. The practitioner should then fill in the treatment preferences—such as arch shape, bracket selection, and arch wire selection—for this specific case. The treatment plan and documentation can then be uploaded to the FTP server of the company. The company transfers the PVS impressions or the stereolithographic (STL) files of the intraoral scan into a digital dental model. The technician will perform the segmentation of the dental crowns for the initial setup model (called T1). Then the setup of the dental crowns is made in the dental lab to simulate the planned treatment result (called T2). For this setup, the position of the lower dentition into the scanned alveolar bone 4 mm below the gingival, the so-called mantrough, will be used to position the teeth in the alveolar bone ridge of the mandible [7]. The finished setup of the dental crowns in the mandibular arch will be used as a template for the setup of the dentition in the maxillary arch (Figure 5.8). The differences in distances between the dental crowns in setup T1 and T2 will be registered and shown on the computer monitor. A "grid" can be used to evaluate the symmetry of T1 and T2. If interproximal reduction has been applied during the of the setup (T2), this will be indicated. Of course, the documentation of this patient—such as an OPT, headplate, CBCT, and intra- and extraoral images—will be used for setup fabrication (Figure 5.9).

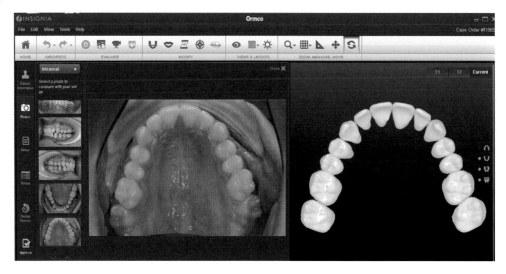

Figure 5.8 Original maxillary arch and a setup.
Company: Ormco.

The position of the upper incisors, possible profile changes, and the design of an ideal smile arch will get special attention in the setup. Evaluation of the facial photographs, facial scan, and the video of the patient during smiling can be used to evaluate the actual "smile line" of the patient during function (Figure 5.10). Occlusal contacts and the occlusion as planned in T2 can be evaluated in the setup, by superimposition and clipping the images.

The setup (T2) will be transferred to the orthodontic office by email for evaluation. The orthodontist can indicate corrections to the lab by mail, and can use the setup software provided by Ormco to correct

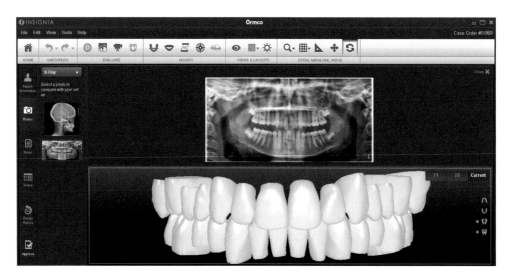

Figure 5.9 The use of an OPT and a setup.
Company: Ormco.

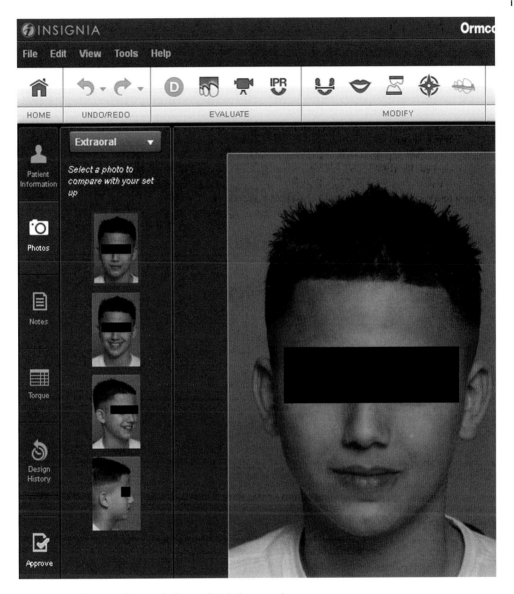

Figure 5.10 Evaluation of the smile line on facial photographs.
Company: Ormco.

the suggested setup in their own computer (T3).

In the suresmile system, the lab technician will, similar to the Insignia system, use the software of that company (which is available online) to correct the initial tooth position after segmentation of the dental crowns on the digital dental model, and, if available, segmentation of the dentition on the CBCT will be performed.

As the suresmile software is available in the Cloud, both the dental technician and the treating doctor are able to correct the setup.

Showing the setup to the patient, the dentist, and the maxillofacial surgeon

After approval or correction of the digital setup for the planned treatment by the orthodontist, the treatment plan will be presented to the patient (and, if indicated, to the referring dentist or the maxillofacial surgeon). As the majority of the appliances and procedures which can be used during treatment can be digitally designed, a realistic overview of the treatment plan, appliances, and the mechanics and interventions which will be used during treatment can be presented. Animations (movies) will show the changes in tooth position from the initial dentition and the setup. Changes in facial appearance, which may be caused by the suggested treatment, will also be discussed. Of course, the outcome of treatment should be a functional and aesthetic, stable result, which corresponds to the desire of the individual patient (Figure 5.11).

After acceptance of the treatment plan, the practitioner will suggest the type of orthodontic appliances which could be used for treatment.

When the practitioner and the patient agree on the appliances and the costs of orthodontic treatment, the same software and the same files used for treatment planning can now be used to design the appliances.

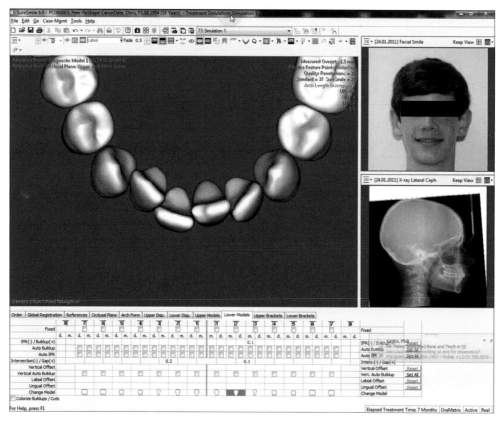

Figure 5.11 Evaluation of the dentition and the digital documentation. Company: OraMetrix.

These digital workflow systems allow excellent communication between patients and clinicians. In addition, appliances can be more accurately fabricated to clinician preferences owing to feedback loops within the digital workflow process.

References

1 Müller-Hartwich, R., Jost-Brinkmann, P.G., and Schubert, K. (2016) Precision of implementing virtual setups for orthodontic treatment using CAD/CAM-fabricated custom archwires. *J. Orofac. Orthop.*, **77** (1), 1–8.

2 Lee, R.J., Pham, J., Weissheimer, A., and Tong, H. (2015) Generating an ideal virtual setup with three-dimensional crowns and roots. *J. Clin. Orthod.*, **49** (11), 696–700.

3 Barreto, M.S., Faber, J., Vogel, C.J., and Araujo, T.M. (2016) Reliability of digital orthodontic setups. *Angle Orthod.*, **86** (2), 255–259.

4 Fabels, L.N. and Nijkamp, P.G. (2014) Interexaminer and intraexaminer reliabilities of 3-dimensional orthodontic digital setups. *Am. J. Orthod. Dentofacial Orthop.*, **146** (6), 806–811.

5 Im, J., Cha, J.Y., Lee, K.J., *et al.* (2014) Comparison of virtual and manual tooth setups with digital and plaster models in extraction cases. *Am. J. Orthod. Dentofacial Orthop.*, **145** (4), 434–442.

6 Farronato, G., Giannini, L., Galbiati, G., *et al.* (2014) Verification of the reliability of the three-dimensional virtual presurgical orthodontic diagnostic protocol. *J. Craniofac. Surg.*, **25** (6), 2013–2016.

7 Andreiko, C. (1994) DDS, MS, on the Elan and Orthos Systems. *J. Clin. Orthod.* **28** (8), 459–468.

6

Custom Appliance Design

K. Hero Breuning

Introduction

Once the patient has accepted a specific treatment plan, orthodontic appliances needed for the planned tooth movement can be selected and designed. For efficient tooth movement a selection of removable, functional, fixed buccal brackets, fixed lingual brackets, or aligners can be used. These days, the use of CAD/CAM procedures in dentistry enables the clinician to customize most of the traditionally used standard orthodontic appliances. Virtual design and the fabrication of custom orthodontic appliances should be used to optimize these appliances for a more effective treatment. A range of dental devices and orthodontic and surgical appliances can now be designed on the virtual patient setup [1]. For the design and fabrication of custom appliances the stereolithographic (STL) files of the digital dental setup representing the accepted treatment plan and dedicated software are used to design dental, orthodontic, and surgical appliances, as needed [2].

Custom design of orthodontic appliances

For orthodontists, Herbst appliances, rapid palatal expansion appliances, twin block appliances, and, for surgeons and dentists, splints for implant placement and surgical splints ("wafers") can be designed and fabricated in an almost total digital workflow [3]. The practitioner should fill in a lab prescription sheet to indicate the requirements for appliances selected for treatment of a specific patient. This lab prescription file should contain all information for the design and fabrication of the appliance and should be sent via Internet to a secure digital portal of the dental lab. In a digital workflow, the STL files of a recent digital dental model should also be transferred to the safe (ftp) site of the dental lab. The technician will then design the appliances, and this design will be returned to the practitioner to be reviewed (Figure 6.1 and Figure 6.2). Ideally, the practitioner should be able to correct or finalize this design. Although most clinicians will outsource the designing of appliances because it takes time and experience to work with the software programs, some practitioners would like to be able to design the appliances themselves or like to have a possibility to control the design of the appliances. If both the lab technician and the orthodontist use the same software program and digital files, they will correct any planned design.

Currently, some labs will send a digital file to the practitioner which contains an image of the setup, in a portable document format (pdf) file, which can be reviewed (but not changed), with a pdf viewer. The orthodontist

Digital Planning and Custom Orthodontic Treatment, First Edition. Edited by K. Hero Breuning and Chung H. Kau.
© 2017 John Wiley & Sons, Inc. Published 2017 by John Wiley & Sons, Inc.

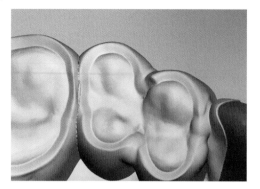

Figure 6.1 Design for three-dimensional printed bands.
Company: Ortholab.

has to indicate the changes required, and send this to the lab technician to actually change this design.

Custom design of aligners

Orthodontic treatment with clear aligners ("invisible orthodontics") started with the introduction of these appliances by Align Technology, Inc., which sells the "Invisalign" aligners. After uploading the prescription

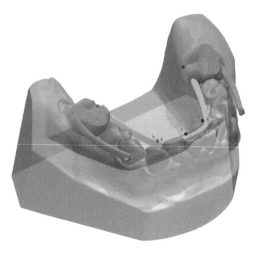

Figure 6.2 Design for a printed Herbst appliance.
Company: 3Shape.

sheet, the digital documentation, and the digital dental models to the website of Invisalign, or one of the many other companies that design and fabricate aligners nowadays, the dental lab can make a setup according to the presented treatment plan. This setup, made by the dental technician, will then be returned to the practitioner to be reviewed. The practitioner should evaluate the setup and indicate the changes needed. After final approval of the setup, the total tooth movement planned is divided into steps. These steps represent the maximum amount of tooth movement which can be achieved with one specific aligner. As an example of limits applied in orthodontics for changing the tip, rotation, or angulation of the dentition with aligners, the tooth moving limit per aligner tray can be set to, for example, 2.5 degrees. For extrusion, intrusion and linear movement of teeth the limit per aligner can be set to 0.25 mm. The amount of printed models and aligners needed for each specific case can then be calculated. Because some tooth movements with aligners are not really possible without increasing the retention between the aligner and the tooth surface, attachments can be designed and transferred with an indirect bonding tray to the dentition so that these attachments can be attached to the actual surface of the tooth. Innovations in aligner treatment, such as the use of "friction pads" as an alternative for the attachments and a combination of a wide range of flexibility of aligners, and a combination of aligners used during daytime and more ridged aligners used at night, have improved the results of aligner treatment [4, 5]. Some companies, such as Ortho Caps, include a planned refinement of the original treatment plan during treatment, and a progress impression or progress scan should be used to make a progress setup and to fabricate progress aligners. Printing of aligners on printed dental models, as an alternative to the traditional fabrication of aligners with sheets, is

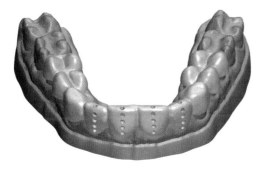

Figure 6.3 Design for a printed splint. Company: 3Shape.

now possible (Figure 6.3). The use of aligners in combination with fixed orthodontic appliances or aligners used to finish treatment after early removal of fixed appliances (hybrid appliances) will increase the use of aligners for tooth correction [6, 7]. Recent software programs, such as 3Shape's Ortho-Analyser and Orchestrate, can be an alternative for Invisalign software. Current fabrication processes can be used to make a setup for aligner fabrication in the dental lab of choice. The design and fabrication of a set of aligners can now also be done in the orthodontic clinic itself (Figure 6.4).

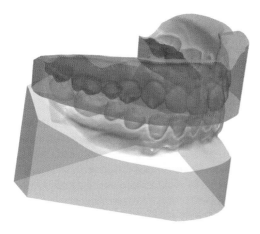

Figure 6.4 Design for a printed positioner. Company: 3Shape.

Virtual bracket placement of standard brackets

Both the initial setup of the dentition and the final setup, which simulates the position of the dentition at the end of orthodontic treatment, can be used for virtual bracket positioning [8–10]. Dedicated software, such as OrthoCAD, suresmile, OnyxCeph, or Ortho-Analyser, can be used to virtually position scanned orthodontic brackets and tubes from a library of scanned standard fixed appliances onto the dental crowns (Figure 6.5). If the brackets are positioned on the final setup, which will increase the efficiency of bracket placement, this bracket position has to be transferred by the software to the dentition of the initial digital model (Figure 6.6).

This virtual bracket positioning process should increase bracket bonding accuracy and reduce the need for wire bending and bracket repositioning during orthodontic treatment, which should finally reduce treatment time and improve the outcome of orthodontic treatment. To further increase the efficiency of an orthodontic fixed appliance system, without increasing the costs of the appliances, some software programs, such as OnyxCeph, can be used to virtually position a series of different standard buccal and lingual brackets (depending on the need for increased or reduced torque values) on the digitized dentition. The use of a selection of bracket prescriptions for each specific case should increase the efficiency of the straight wire system used. A custom bracket base can then be used to improve the fit of the bracket base of the standard bracket used and the dentition. For lingual systems the combination of standard brackets with individual bases was introduced several decades ago. A combination of a custom bracket base and custom wires was recently introduced by the OraMetrix company: the "Fusion" system.

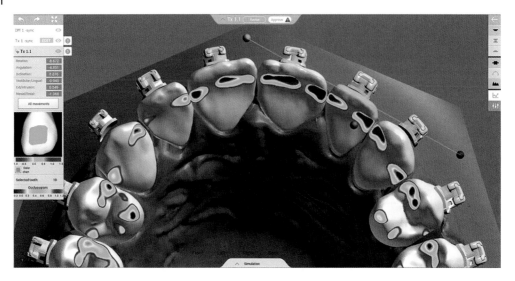

Figure 6.5 Virtually placed buccal brackets.
Company: Exceed-Ortho.

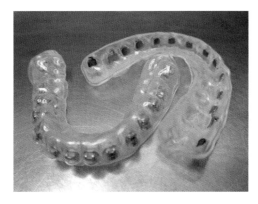

Figure 6.6 Complete indirect bonding trays.
Company: Image Instruments.

Fully customized orthodontic appliance systems

As complete customized orthodontic appliance systems such as custom brackets, custom bracket bases, and custom tubes—including transpalatal arches, headgear tubes, rapid palatal expanders, and attachments for Herbst appliances—can now be designed according to the wishes of the orthodontist and the requirements of each specific case, the use of fully customized orthodontic treatment with a full range of appliance systems is now possible. The first custom wire system commercially available and now widely used in orthodontics was the suresmile system, made by the OraMetrix company in the US. The company started to sell "finishing wires" designed by computer software on the digital images of a scanned dentition during treatment. After fabrication of the setup, the wires with a dimension, flexibility, and force value as has been selected by the practitioner are bent in three dimensions by a wire-bending robot and can be used to finish a case. Depending on the requirements of the case, extra torque can be ordered in specific wires to compensate for the "bracket play" and side effects of the biomechanical system used.

Specific CAD/CAM-designed custom orthodontic treatment systems (a combination of custom wires, custom brackets, and a segmented indirect bonding tray), such as Insignia by Ormco for buccal brackets (Figure 6.7), and custom lingual fixed appliance systems—such as Incognito™ by 3M, Harmony™ by American Orthodontics, and

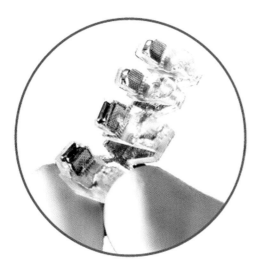

Figure 6.7 Segmented indirect bonding trays. Company: Ormco.

eBrace/eLock by the Guangzhou Riton Biomaterial Co for lingual brackets (Figure 6.8)—are now also commercially available [11–13].

For all custom fixed appliance systems, indirect bonding trays or jigs should be designed to transfer the custom appliances to the dentition. The actual implementation of the indirect bonding trays (full arch or a tray divided into pieces can be selected by the practitioner. These systems should be used with a set of custom orthodontic wires as prescribed by the orthodontist.

Custom design of orthodontic retention appliances

Orthodontic retention appliances—such as removable retainers, tooth positioners, retention wires, surgical splints, and mandibular repositioning appliances for treating sleep apnea and snoring, for orthodontic patients—can now also be designed and printed three-dimensionally with dedicated software. Some printed appliances need to be post-processed, for example to assemble printed parts. If physical dental models are needed, printed dental models can be used [14].

Conclusion

Utilizing state-of-the art hardware and software platforms, custom appliance design allows control over appliance design and fabrication. Indirect bonding is required to transfer the custom appliances to the dentition of the patient.

This indirect bonding process will increase the accurate placement of the appliances, while some of the pitfalls commonly associated with the conventional bonding process will be avoided. Computer-assisted procedures have long been seen as advantageous in other medical branches as well as in orthodontic aligner therapy. Computerized treatment planning and bracket positioning and the use of custom appliances are extending this concept to the area of fixed appliances. As more software programs become available and the fabrication process of custom brackets and wires becomes more affordable, these customized appliance systems will be used a great deal more. This increased use of custom orthodontic appliances will reduce the costs of these appliance systems.

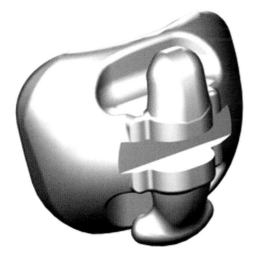

Figure 6.8 Design for a custom lingual bracket. Company: Guangzhou Riton Biomaterial Co.

References

1 Al Mortadi, N., Jones, Q., Eggbeer, D., *et al.* (2015) Fabrication of a resin appliance with alloy components using digital technology without an analog impression. *Am. J. Orthod. Dentofacial Orthop.*, **148** (5), 862–867.

2 Salmi, M., Paloheimo, K.S., Tuomi, J., *et al.* (2013) A digital process for additive manufacturing of occlusal splints: a clinical pilot study. *J. R. Soc. Interface.*, doi: 10.1098/rsif.2013.0203.

3 van der Meer, W.J., Vissink, A., and Ren, Y. (2016) Full 3-dimensional digital workflow for multicomponent dental appliances: a proof of concept. *J. Am. Dent. Assoc.*, **147** (4), 288–291.

4 Javidi, H. and Graham, E. (2015) Clear aligners for orthodontic treatment? *Evid. Based. Dent.*, **16** (4), 111.

5 Hennessy, J. and Al-Awadhi, E.A. (2016) Clear aligners generations and orthodontic tooth movement. *J. Orthod.*, **8**, 1–9.

6 Azaripour, A., Weusmann, J., Mahmoodi, B., *et al.* (2015) Braces versus Invisalign®: gingival parameters and patients' satisfaction during treatment: a cross-sectional study. *BMC Oral Health*, **15**, 69.

7 Han, J.Y. (2015) A comparative study of combined periodontal and orthodontic treatment with fixed appliances and clear aligners in patients with periodontitis. *J. Periodontal Implant. Sci.*, **45** (6), 193–204.

8 Suárez, C. and Vilar, T. (2010) The effect of constant height bracket placement on marginal ridge levelling using digitized models. *Eur. J. Orthod.*, **32** (1), 100–105.

9 Nojima, L.I., Araújo, A.S., and Alves Júnior, M. (2015) Indirect orthodontic bonding: a modified technique for improved efficiency and precision. *Dental Press J. Orthod.*, **20** (3), 109–117.

10 Flores, T., Mayoral, J.R., Giner, L., and Puigdollers, A. (2015) Comparison of enamel-bracket bond strength using direct- and indirect-bonding techniques with a self-etching ion releasing S-PRG filler. *Dent. Mater. J.*, **34** (1), 41–47.

11 Menini, A., Cozzani, M., Sfondrini, M.F., *et al.* (2014) A 15-month evaluation of bond failures of orthodontic brackets bonded with direct versus indirect bonding technique: a clinical trial. *Prog. Orthod.*, **30**(15), 70.

12 Brown, M.W., Koroluk, L., Ko, C.C., *et al.* (2015) Effectiveness and efficiency of a CAD/CAM orthodontic bracket system. *Am. J. Orthod. Dentofacial Orthop.*, **148** (6), 1067–1074.

13 Kwon, S.Y., Kim, Y., Ahn, H.W., *et al.* (2014) Computer-aided designing and manufacturing of lingual fixed orthodontic appliance using 2D/3D registration software and rapid prototyping. *Int. J. Dent.*, doi: 10.1155/2014/164164.

14 Wolf, M., Schumacher, P., Jäger, F., *et al.* (2015) Novel lingual retainer created using CAD/CAM technology: evaluation of its positioning accuracy. *J. Orofac. Orthop.*, **76** (2), 164–174.

7

Custom Appliance Fabrication and Transfer

K. Hero Breuning

Introduction

The fabrication and transfer of the custom orthodontic appliances should be accurate and requires an efficient workflow [1]. For the CAD/CAM processes, the (STL) files of the digital dental setup will represent the design of the appliances, and dedicated software can then be used by three-dimensional (3D) printers and wire-bending robots to fabricate the appliances. Three-dimensional printed processes can be used to print physical dental models in acrylic material (Figure 7.1). These printed models can be used for the traditional fabrication methods of removable and functional orthodontic appliances (Figure 7.2).

These printed models are also needed to assemble the different parts of the appliances after 3D printing in the dental lab with laser sintering of printed and prefabricated parts. For orthodontic appliances, such as rapid expansion devices or Herbst appliances expansion screws or the prefabricated parts of the Herbst Appliances, have to be assembled to the printed parts of the appliance in a dental lab [2].Although virtual articulators can be used during the designing process (Ortho-Analyser), the use of physical articulators can still be required. Currently, there is a range of 3D printers available for printing physical dental models. The prices of the 3D printers have been reduced and the quality of the printed dental models of most 3D printers is sufficient for orthodontic use. We evaluated at the University in Nijmegen, the accuracy of printed digital dental models from the files of an intraoral scanner and concluded that the printed models with a base or a bar between the molars are, compared with the "gold standard" plaster model, accurate and can be used for appliance fabrication in orthodontics (Figure 7.3). However, we found that the transversal distances between the cuspids and molars on printed models without a base or a connecting bar between the molars were significantly and clinically smaller for the 3D printer used when only a "horseshoe" model (no base or bar) was printed.

Aligner fabrication

A series of printed models of the same patient can be used to fabricate a series of clear aligners ("invisible braces") to move the teeth gradually into the desired direction (Figure 7.4). After printing a series of physical models representing the steps between the original position of the dental crowns and the setup, clear vacuum formed flexible appliances can be made on the dental models with vacuum machines. As an alternative, the aligners can be printed in 3D without the need for a physical dental model [2]. A series

Digital Planning and Custom Orthodontic Treatment, First Edition. Edited by K. Hero Breuning and Chung H. Kau.
© 2017 John Wiley & Sons, Inc. Published 2017 by John Wiley & Sons, Inc.

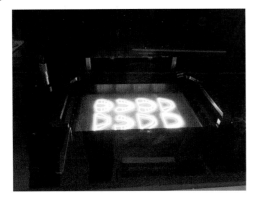

Figure 7.1 Printing of dental models.
Company: Orthoproof.

of clear aligners can then be used to gradually move the dentition into the desired direction. Recently, 3D printed aligners in flexible material have become available as an alternative to the vacuum formed sheets.

Custom orthodontic brackets and tubes

Different materials can be selected for the fabrication of custom fixed appliances. The

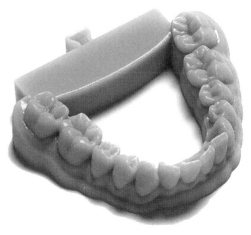

Figure 7.3 "Horseshoe" printed model with bar for aligner fabrication.
Company: Orthoproof.

custom Incognito lingual braces are printed in wax and then transferred to a gold alloy. The base of the Harmony lingual brackets and the Insignia buccal brackets is printed in a metal alloy, and for the eBrace and eLock systems a range of different materials is available for 3D printing of the brackets and bracket base [3]. A "copy" of the Incognito brackets

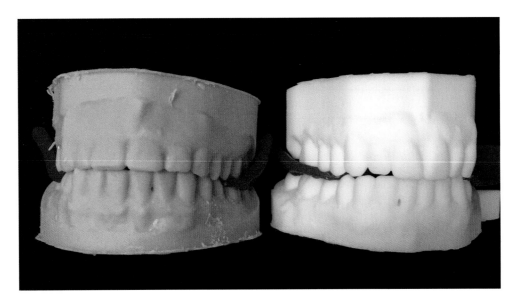

Figure 7.2 Printed dental models.
Company: Orthoproof.

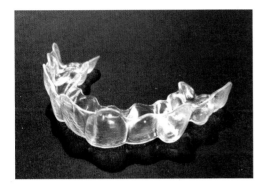

Figure 7.4 Example of a printed aligner.
Company: Orthoproof.

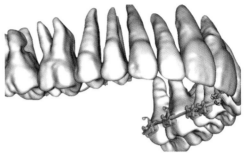

Figure 7.6 A customized lingual bracket system with computer bend wires.
Company: OraMetrix.

(brackets and bracket base made of a gold alloy) is now available (Figure 7.5).

Custom wire fabrication

As an alternative for wire bending, a set of custom wires with a selected diameter, shape, elastic properties, and tooth moving force values, according to the prescription of the orthodontist, can be bent by a wire-bending robot. The company OraMetrix (suresmile) started this wire-bending service some decades ago. Research has shown that the use of custom wires to finish orthodontic treatment will reduce treatment time and can be used to improve the treated result [4]. Some custom systems, such as Insignia and Fusion, use individual wires with first order

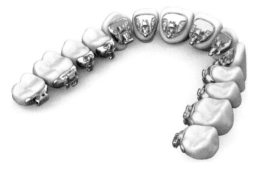

Figure 7.5 Custom lingual brackets with casted or printed bracket base.
Company: Guangzhou Riton Biomaterial Co.

steps only for orthodontic treatment with buccal brackets (Figure 7.6). Other custom appliance systems—such as Incognito, Harmony, eBrace/eLock, and others—will provide custom wires with first-, second-, and third-order bends, depending on the requirements of the case for lingual orthodontic treatment [5, 6].

Fabrication of orthodontic transfer appliances

For transfer of the custom orthodontic fixed appliances to the dentition, physical dental models can be printed with 3D printers. In the OrthoCAD, OnyxCeph, and Exceed software systems, the virtually planned position of the brackets will be indicated on the printed models. In the dental lab, the technician has to position the selected brackets on this dental model to fabricate the trays with a vacuum tray on a machine, such as the Biostar machine. As an alternative to vacuum formed trays, soft silicone material and a second layer of harder silicon material can be used. Special materials have been developed for fabrication of this indirect bonding tray, such as Emiluma™ and Lumaloc™ made by Opal Orthodontics.

An alternative method to make the indirect bonding devices can be to print the trays or transfer jigs with dedicated 3D printers or fabricate these trays with milling

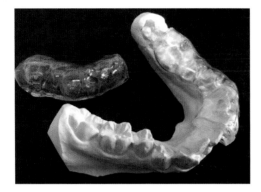

Figure 7.7 Segmented indirect bonding tray for the mandibular arch.
Company: Orthoproof.

machines. To reduce bonding failures, some orthodontists like to segment the bonding trays. The bonding appliances can be segmented according to the wishes of the clinician (Figure 7.7).

Transfer of custom fixed appliances to the dentition

To transfer the planned position of the prefabricated and custom orthodontic buccal and lingual fixed appliances to the actual dentition of the patient, a bonding tray or bonding jigs should be used. Transparency of the trays and jigs will allow the use of light cure adhesive. As large bonding pads are used for customized lingual brackets, a dual cure adhesive (both chemical and light cured adhesive) can be required. Different bonding materials and protocols are presented for bonding the brackets [7, 8].

The bonding procedure

Proper isolation and saliva contamination are critical to successful bonding. Cheek retractors, absorbent pads (dry angles), and a high-speed evacuator are highly recommended. For this bonding procedure, a Nola System—total dry field system or Kerr Corporation's Optiview lip retractors combined with dry angles and cotton rolls—can be used to effectively avoid moisture contamination during bonding (Figure 7.8 and Figure 7.9). Enamel tooth surfaces are first cleaned, rinsed, and then dried. Then, the surface will usually be prepared for bonding with a 37% phosphoric acid etching gel. A bonding agent

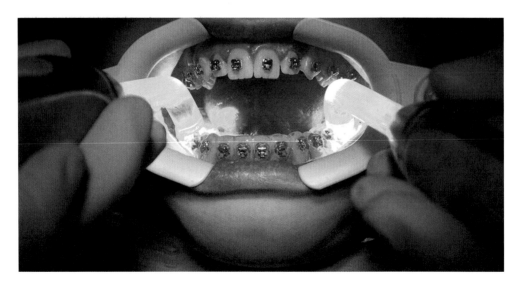

Figure 7.8 Indirect bonding procedure: a dry field system.
Company: Great Lakes Orthodontics.

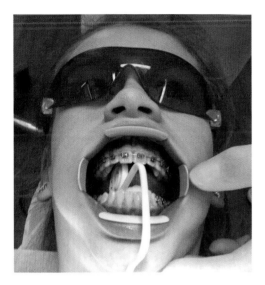

Figure 7.9 Alternative dry field system.
Company: Kerr Corporation.

is then applied to each tooth and the adhesive is distributed and firmly pressed into the bracket pad. The makers of some customized bonding systems suggest one sandblasts the enamel before bonding, but we suggest doing this only for restored teeth or after bracket failure. Special preparation for dental fillings, gold surfaces, and ceramics restorations may be needed. Reduction of bonding steps

can be achieved if an etching plus primer combination is used. If the tooth surface is ready for bonding, the bonding trays or jigs are seated and the bracket adhesive is light-cured. Nowadays, chemical curing of adhesive is only used for lingual appliances. The light curing starts in the region of molars and then the tray is stabilized in the central incisor region by curing the incisal brackets. After complete adhesive curing, the dual layer or single layer trays are carefully removed by peeling the tray from the dentition. After removal, a scaler or explorer is used to check for excess of adhesive and any excess bonding material is removed. Dental floss should be used to check the presence of adhesive between the contact points.

The potential advantages offered by this indirect bracket positioning and bonding method are considerable. From a clinical standpoint, optimized bracket placement can provide gains during the total process of initial alignment, arch correction, and finishing. The bonding of second molar tubes at the start of treatment, which is more easy if indirect bonding is used, will increase the efficiency of orthodontic mechanics. As far as office management is concerned, the time needed for bonding can be significantly

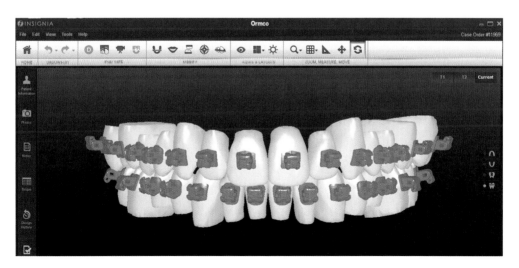

Figure 7.10 Digital planning of bracket position.
Company: Ormco.

shorter for indirect bonding compared to direct bonding of brackets. This indirect bonding procedure will also be more comfortable for the patient. As many steps in the orthodontic office are now delegated to assistants, an indirect bonding procedure can be delegated to trained staff members, requiring minimal or no doctor time. The orthodontist should review the bracket and tube positions during treatment planning and not during the actual bonding procedure (Figure 7.10). In our opinion, indirect bonding after digital planning of the bracket positon method can make orthodontic treatment more predictable, with fewer re-bracketing and wire-bending appointments necessary.

Overall, a bonding system to transfer the brackets and tubes from the digitally planned positon to the dentition provides a solution to one of the key issues in most orthodontic clinics. Because several steps in this bonding procedure are sensitive to failures, the fabrication of the bonding trays or jigs should best be outsourced to a dental lab.

Rebonding brackets and tubes

The original transfer tray can be cut into pieces for rebonding of several brackets or for

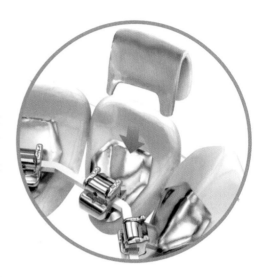

Figure 7.11 Rebonding jig for lingual brackets. Company: American Orthodontics.

rebonding individual brackets. For rebonding of incisal and cuspid lingual brackets for custom lingual bracket systems, bracket positioning jigs should be provided (Figure 7.11).

When the bracket pads are completely devoid of any previous adhesive residue, there is no need to have them reconditioned. If a customized bracket base of adhesive is present, extra preparation steps before bonding, such as sandblasting or the use of a primer, are required.

References

1 van Noort, R. (2012) The future of dental devices is digital. *Dent. Mater.*, **28** (1), 3–12.

2 Fayyaz Ahamed, S., Apros Kanna, A.S., and Vijaya Kumar, R.K. (2015) 3D printed orthodontic auxiliaries. *J. Clin. Orthod.*, **49** (5), 337–341.

3 Martorelli, M., Gerbino, S., Giudice, M., and Ausiello, P. (2013) A comparison between customized clear and removable orthodontic appliances manufactured using RP and CNC techniques. *Dent. Mater.*, **29** (2), e1–e10.

4 Kwon, S.Y., Kim, Y., Ahn, H.W., *et al.* (2014) Computer-aided designing and manufacturing of lingual fixed orthodontic appliance using 2D/3D registration software and rapid prototyping. *Int. J. Dent.*, doi: 10.1155/2014/164164.

5 Saxe, A.K., Louie, L.J., and Mah, J. (2010) Efficiency and effectiveness of SureSmile. *World J. Orthod.*, **11** (1): 16–22.

6 Grauer, D., Wiechmann, D., Heymann, G.C., and Swift, E.J. Jr. (2012) Computer-aided

design/computer-aided manufacturing technology in customized orthodontic appliances. *J. Esthet. Restor. Dent.*, **24** (1), 3–9.

7 Israel, M., Kusnoto, B., Evans, C.A., and Begole, E. (2011) A comparison of traditional and computer-aided bracket

placement methods. *Angle. Orthod.*, **81** (5), 828–835.

8 Castilla, A.E., Crowe, J.J., Moses, J.R., *et al.* (2014) Measurement and comparison of bracket transfer accuracy of five indirect bonding techniques. *Angle. Orthod.*, **84** (4), 607–614.

8

Monitoring of Tooth Movement

Philippe Salah and K. Hero Breuning

Introduction

Once a treatment plan for orthodontics has been made by the orthodontist and agreed by the patient, standard or custom orthodontic appliances are fabricated and positioned on the dentition, tooth movement with removable, fixed buccal, or lingual orthodontic appliances or aligner systems can be started. Effective and optimal tooth movement is needed to achieve the planned change in tooth position. According to published research, the speed of tooth movement will be different for each individual and depends on the orthodontic mechanics used. The orthodontist will use optimal mechanical systems for tooth movement (wires or aligners), and during treatment control visits at certain intervals are scheduled. These control visits should be scheduled according to the need to change (or reactivate) the mechanical system used, to optimize tooth movement. But as tooth movement for an individual patient is not registered, optimal planning of control visits is not possible. Activation of the tooth movement system (changing of the wires or aligners), will not always lead to faster tooth movement, because of the occurrence of hyalinization in the periodontal ligament after activation. So consequent monitoring of tooth movement at planned intervals could be used to optimize the timing of control visits. This monitoring of tooth

movement will also help the orthodontist and the patient to visualize whether the actual tooth movement ensures the achievement of the planned treatment goal. As healthcare evolves, healthcare facilities are staying almost continually in touch with their patients and offer them more customized patient care. This visualization will also be a motivational tool for the patients, their families, and friends.

Monitoring of tooth movement can be achieved by analyzing progress intraoral scans with dedicated software programs, such as Ortho-Analyser (Figure 8.1) [1]. During control visits, a progress scan can be made and superimposed on the initial scan to reveal the differences in tooth position. A disadvantage of this type of monitoring is that the patient has to visit the orthodontic office to make an intraoral scan. Alternatively, an extra oral photograph can be used to correct the "smile line" (Figure 8.2) or a second cone beam computer tomography (CBCT) radiograph can be made to evaluate the tooth position (Figure 8.3) and the jaw positon after a surgical correction (Figure 8.4). Specific software programs can be used to superimpose the CBCT radiographs and facial scans (Figure 8.5). A "progress setup" can then be made to correct the tooth position according to the progress documentation, and fabrication of a "finishing wire" or "finishing aligners" can then be used to correct the dentition.

Digital Planning and Custom Orthodontic Treatment, First Edition. Edited by K. Hero Breuning and Chung H. Kau.
© 2017 John Wiley & Sons, Inc. Published 2017 by John Wiley & Sons, Inc.

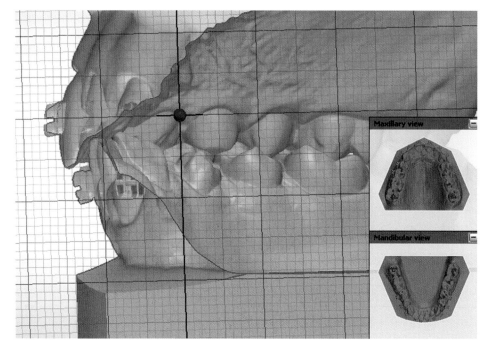

Figure 8.1 Analysis of a progress dental scan using the "clipping" function. Company: 3Shape.

A disadvantage of these monitoring systems is that the patient will not be able to actually see treatment progress at home.

Recently, a new monitoring system for orthodontics was introduced by a company called Dental Monitoring. This company, based in Paris, will remotely monitor the patient's tooth movements and treatment progress using the patient's smartphone. An essential part of Dental Monitoring's system is a custom cheek retractor which will be used every time the patient takes pictures with their smartphone. This cheek retractor was specially designed to help the patient take quality pictures with ease. They have visual markings that are important in calibrating the pictures taken (Figure 8.6).

Workflow for the dental monitoring system

The Dental Monitoring website allows the orthodontist to create new patient files, upload their three-dimensional (3D) impressions, view the photos the patient has uploaded, and monitor their treatment. Orthodontists have to go to the website to register as a Dental Monitoring user. They will then get a username and password by mail within two days. On the secured doctor site, patients can be added. The orthodontist should fill in the information of a specific patient. The orthodontist and patient will then get their activation code to register on the Dental Monitoring app: available for Apple and Android users for free. Then the patient should download the Dental Monitoring app. Before monitoring begins, the orthodontist has to provide recent, accurate plaster models, PVS impressions, or intraoral scans of a specific patient. The transport of the models or impressions with UPS is included in the fee. The company will then scan the plaster models or impressions to get a digital dental model which will be used as a reference for treatment monitoring. Requirements for the impression are: the

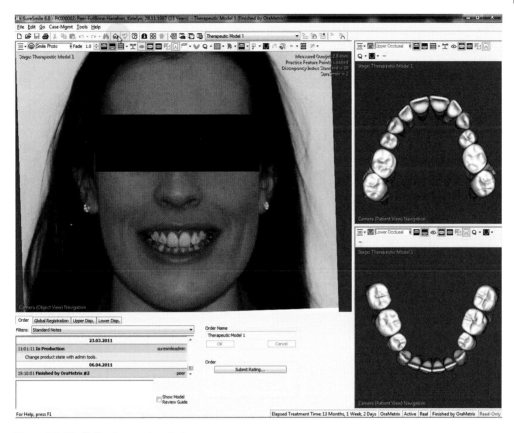

Figure 8.2 "Smile line" correction during treatment.
Company: OraMetrix.

impression can be taken while the patient is wearing braces but must not contain holes. Removal of the wires before impression taking will improve the quality of the impressions. For an intraoral scan, removal

of the wires is usually not necessary, but the impression cannot contain any artifacts so the orthodontist should ensure that there are no defects or distortions in the impression or the digital scan. The costs of transport, the

Figure 8.3 Evaluation of the tooth position on a cone beam computer tomography radiograph.
Company: OraMetrix.

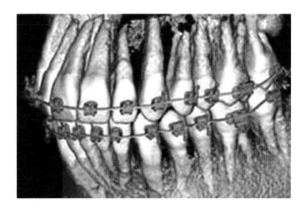

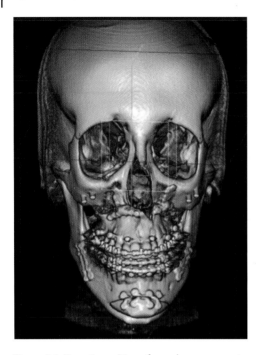

Figure 8.4 Superimposition of cone beam computer tomography radiograph's after jaw surgery.
Company: Dolphin Imaging & Management Solutions.

scanning of the model, or the impressions can be reduced if the orthodontist transfers the models or impressions with their own desktop scanner or uses an intraoral scanner. If the orthodontist has asked one of Dental Monitoring's partner labs to scan the impressions, the lab will upload the files. The webpage should be used to upload the files. Currently, the digital data (stereolithographic (STL) files) from several intraoral scanners are accepted: the Trios scanner (3Shape), iTero, and the Carestream Dental scanner. Of course, the scan should be very accurate and the files must be in STL format. A bite registration such as a wax bite or an intraoral scan of the molars and incisors in occlusion is also required.

For each set of files, the date the impression was taken has to be filled in and the type of treatment planned and the type of monitoring required for the specific case should

be indicated. In 2016, the 3Shape company created a seamless integration between the intraoral scans of the Trios intraoral scanner and the Dental Monitoring Company. This integration enables orthodontists using the intraoral scanner to send digital impressions directly to the Dental Monitoring platform with just a click. The 3Shape Trios integration now gives orthodontists using these solutions an easy, accurate, and fast tool for monitoring the treatment progress. Orthodontists using 3Shape's Trios can select Dental Monitoring from the list of integrated solution providers within the intraoral scanner's software. From there, the orthodontist just needs to click to send the Trios digital impression and case information directly to the Dental Monitoring platform. Because the digital impression becomes the first reference point in defining the baseline tooth position as well as a benchmark for all future calculations made by the application, it makes the accuracy of the initial intraoral scan paramount. The smooth integration between Trios STL files and the platform will make it much easier for orthodontists and patients to take advantage of the innovative platform. The uploaded files will be quality controlled and analyzed upon reception by the Dental Monitoring company. In most cases the files will be suitable to be used, and the company will be able to proceed directly to their analysis. If the files are found to be insufficiently accurate to be superimposed on earlier digital dental models, the orthodontist will receive an alert message on their dashboard of their personal page on the Dental Monitoring website and will be informed of what action is needed to solve these problems. When the issues reported have been rectified, the orthodontist can submit the new files.

The orthodontist has to specify the monitoring type to the dental lab: is this patient in observation? Will an early interception treatment be started or is the patient in active treatment? If treatment has finished, impressions or an intraoral scan of the finished

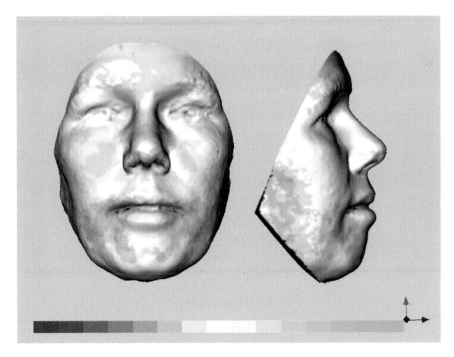

Figure 8.5 Superimposition of facials scans with a "color distance map."
Company: 3dMD.

dentition can be used for fabrication of a finished digital dental model. The specialists at the Dental Monitoring lab need the information of the status of the treatment phase to tailor the alerts the orthodontist or the patient will receive. For pre-treatment monitoring, the usual frequency of each photo exam is every three months. During treatment, a photo exam is scheduled every two weeks, and during post-treatment monitoring, one photo exam is scheduled every

two months. The patient will get regular reminders by mail to make the planned series of photographs or a video of the dentition and send them to Dental Monitoring.

Every photo exam or video should be uploaded to Dental Monitoring's server and will be analyzed by dental specialists, including supervision of a qualified orthodontist. If there are important changes in the patient's dentition while they're being monitored, for example a progress intraoral scan or a

Figure 8.6 Cheek retraction device with markers.
Company: Dental Monitoring.

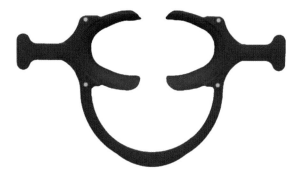

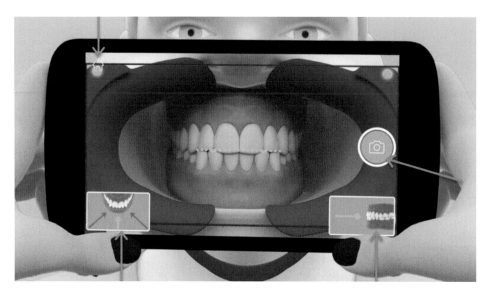

Figure 8.7 The "smartphone" used to make a series of pictures of the dentition.
Company: Dental Monitoring.

finishing scan has been made, this scan can be uploaded to DM and this new 3D model can then be used as a reference.

The fee for this service will depend on the number of monitored patients. Price reductions are automatically applied according to the usage by each specific doctor or clinic. The orthodontist or auxiliary personnel can help the patient to use the app and how to take their first photo set. The patient should take eight to 12 pictures for each photo set (Figure 8.7).

Following the recommendations of the orthodontist, the patients will be notified by email that a new set of photos or a video is required. If the frequency of this procedure should be changed, for instance after the start of treatment or at the start of the monitoring of the retention, the patient will receive a message.

The Dental Monitoring app is compatible with iPhones 4s or later running iOS 7.0 or higher and smartphones running Android 4.0.3 or higher.

The download procedure of the app and the instructions on how to make the required series of photos, and the use of the Dental Monitoring cheek retractor can be best completed in the orthodontist's office. The patient should teach the person who will take the pictures how to do this. Ideally, that second person comes to the orthodontist's office for instruction and to practice this procedure.

Dental Monitoring has created a Demo Mode to help the patient understand how to use the Dental Monitoring app and how to take acceptable pictures. A short video tutorial which clearly shows the steps needed to take optimal pictures is available on Dental Monitoring's website.

Procedure for taking pictures

- Turn the phone sideways to begin taking pictures.
- Prior to each picture, three diagrams will appear on the patient's phone demonstrating the desired orientation.
- The next step is to take the pictures.
- The entire mouth and the retractor must be in the frame.
- Be close enough: the retractor is the external frame of the picture.

- The lips must not cover the gum line.
- The green line on the retractors must be in the center of the pictures.
- The green line shows how widely the mouth should be opened.
- The green line should be aligned with the bottom of the incisors in a closed mouth position.
- For lateral pictures of the dentition, the patient must pull the retractor toward both the right and left sides.
- The pictures must be as perpendicular as possible to the premolars.
- Press the shutter release to make the picture.
- Check if the picture is correct.
- Retake the picture when it is blurry, the green lines are not aligned with the teeth, etc.

When all the pictures are taken, the patient will be taken back to the website's home page, where a message will appear indicating that the series of photos are being sent to Dental Monitoring. As the downloading procedure will be stopped as the application is closed during the uploading procedure, the application should not be closed until all pictures for this session are sent. However, downloading will start again from the point it stopped when the app was reopened.

At the Dental Monitoring lab, analysis of the pictures will be started as soon as possible. The actual position of each tooth will be compared to the initial tooth position and the tooth position registered during earlier digital monitoring of the tooth position with a set of intraoral pictures. Dental Monitoring will provide an analysis of the tooth movement with dedicated computer software and this report will appear four days after the series of photographs are received on the dashboard of the secured Internet site, which is available for each orthodontist.

The report of the analysis shows the actual tooth position which has been compared to the initial tooth position on the digital dental model and series of earlier recorded photographs by computers. In this analysis, the movement of the selected tooth can be evaluated in all directions.

Three-dimensional matching of images and the initial digital dental model is possible and visualizes the actual movement of the dentition in the selected period of time. The rapport of this analysis of tooth movement in 3D includes a graph, showing the tooth movement velocity of each tooth [1–4]. The steeper the slope of this graph, the faster the teeth are moving. Initially, one chart for each type of movement was provided, but now that information is provided with two charts. One chart shows movement of translation, and the other shows movements of rotation in degrees.

Each chart has three graphs corresponding to one specific type of translation or rotation, and any one of these graphs can be separately evaluated. Each type of movement is clearly defined on the graphs, for more precision in the analysis. This means the orthodontist can now compare the actual pictures with the stored digital dental model and with previous registrations of intraoral photographs.

Dental monitoring alerts

If an unexpected situation is detected through the Dental Monitoring algorithm by the company's technicians, the orthodontist will receive an immediate alert on their dashboard, in the "Actions Required" tab. The orthodontist can now easily assess the significance of the alert and review detailed information about the affected teeth and suspect movements reported. Bracket failure, wire failure, and failures of the wire bracket connection are examples of alerts that will be sent to the orthodontist. If the patient agrees, a patient file can be shared with another practitioner, such as the referring dentist or a dental specialist. To share a patient file the other practitioner's email address should be filled in on the website. A email will be sent to the practitioner inviting them to share the files (in a read-only version, if selected).

The orthodontist can decide to send a registration code to the patient's email address. This allows the patient to review the series of images and the overlay of the initial tooth position and the change in tooth position during treatment. Patients will not receive the tooth moving graphs and the alerts sent to the orthodontist during treatment.

Discussion

Both the orthodontists and the patient are interested in the speed of tooth movement. Dental monitoring systems can be used to effectively monitor these tooth movements [5–7]. Today, the orthodontist can show the initial documentation, the planned treatment (a digital dental setup), and maybe even the planned facial outcome. But during treatment, this tooth movement is only visually reviewed by the practitioner, during the scheduled control visits. These monitoring systems have the advantage of showing the speed of tooth movement and the direction of tooth movement during a selected time interval. For the intraoral scan, the patient has to visit the office, but not if they just need to take photographs or videos of their teeth. This can be done anywhere.

After the (easy) process of uploading the photographic images to the Dental Monitoring lab, both the orthodontist and the patient will be able to see how treatment is progressing. A technician and an orthodontist will review each case and, if needed, an alert will be sent to the orthodontist. Depending on the nature of this alert, the orthodontist can decide to email the patient to schedule an appointment to reattach a bracket, change a broken wire, etc. If tooth movement in a specific patient is faster than expected, the orthodontist can observe this in the tooth movement graph. In these cases, a control visit can be scheduled to reactivate the tooth moving mechanics. If tooth movement is still going on, a scheduled control visit could possibly be postponed. So this monitoring of tooth movement will enable individually planned control visits. If the orthodontist has to adapt the treatment mechanics, because undesired tooth movement has been detected, early correction can be planned. The customization of control visits and the early detection of treatment emergencies, such as unplanned tooth movements, can help the orthodontist to finish each case more efficiently. Some digital planning software allows the exportation of the STL files of the planned result after treatment, and in the next future it will be possible not only to compare the actual tooth position with the beginning of treatment but also project the tooth movement needed to reach the planned result on the virtual final setup. An estimation of the time needed to finish treatment could then be added to this monitoring system.

Of course, this monitoring could also be used to register the level of oral hygiene during treatment. Decalcifications can be detected before serious dental decay develops. Preventive measures can be taken.

In our opinion, documenting treatment progress to evaluate the need to correct an initial treatment plan is always required. If an initial CBCT is available, a progress intraoral scan can be used to review the dental crown position, including the roots during treatment. Some software programs can be used to merge the dental crowns and the dentition on the CBCT. So when an initial CBCT is available, the dentition out of this CBCT can be merged with the progress scan of the dental crowns. A new progress CBCT is then possibly not required. In some cases, a progress setup is needed to correct the treatment results achieved during the first phase of orthodontic treatment. After approval of this progress setup, progress appliances, such as progress wires, can be ordered from companies such as the suresmile company. As the quality of the scanned brackets on CBCT radiographs is not accurate because of scattering and the relatively large voxel size of the radiographs taken for orthodontic purposes, super-impositions of scanned brackets and the image of the brackets on the CBCT are often needed to enable custom wire fabrication.

Conclusion

It should be mentioned that at this moment there are no scientific studies showing the accuracy of dental monitoring systems. In the literature, retrospective tooth movement during orthodontic treatment has been evaluated in 3D [5–7]. The accuracy of super-impositions of digital dental models, digital photographs with markers, CBCTs, and facial scans with software programs—such as Maxillim (owned by Medicim), Geomagic (3D Systems), Dolphin (Dolphin Imaging & Management Solutions), and Ortho-Analyser (3Shape)—seem to be clinically accurate. There are currently no studies on the accuracy of the different monitoring system as presented in this chapter. But even if the recorded tooth and jaw movements are not 100% accurate, this monitoring will help both the orthodontist and the patient to visualize and correct the orthodontic treatment, and these processes can be used to register and solve possible complications during orthodontic treatment.

References

1 Cha, B.K., Lee, J.Y., Jost-Brinkmann, P.G., and Yoshida, N. (2007) Analysis of tooth movement in extraction cases using three-dimensional reverse engineering technology. *Eur. J. Orthod.*, **29** (4), 325–331.

2 Choi, J.I., Cha, B.K., Jost-Brinkmann, P.G., *et al.* (2012) Validity of palatal superimposition of 3-dimensional digital models in cases treated with rapid maxillary expansion and maxillary protraction headgear. *Korean J. Orthod.*, **42** (5), 235–241.

3 An, K., Jang, I., Choi, D.S., *et al.* (2015) Identification of a stable reference area for superimposing mandibular digital models. *J. Orofac. Orthop.*, **76** (6), 508–519.

4 Lee, R.J., Pham, J., Choy, M., *et al.* (2014) Monitoring of typodont root movement via crown superimposition of single cone-beam computed tomography and consecutive intraoral scans. *Am. J. Orthod. Dentofacial Orthop.*, **145** (3), 399–409.

5 Lai, E.H., Yao, C.C., Chang, J.Z., *et al.* (2008) Three-dimensional dental model analysis of treatment outcomes for protrusive maxillary dentition: comparison of headgear, miniscrew, and miniplate skeletal anchorage. *Am. J. Orthod. Dentofacial Orthop.*, **134** (5), 636–645.

6 Park, T.J., Lee, S.H., and Lee, K.S. (2012) A method for mandibular dental arch superimposition using 3D cone beam CT and orthodontic 3D digital model. *Korean J. Orthod.*, **42** (4), 169–181.

7 Lee, R.J., Weissheimer, A., Pham, J., *et al.* (2015) Three-dimensional monitoring of root movement during orthodontic treatment. *Am. J. Orthod. Dentofacial Orthop.*, **147** (1), 132–142.

9

Custom Retention after Orthodontic Treatment

K. Hero Breuning

Introduction

After orthodontic tooth movement, prolonged stabilization of the dentition, especially in the incisor and cuspid region, is recommended [1]. In the last decades of the last century, most removable retainers were replaced by fixed lingual retainers because they require less patient compliance and are effective for 24 hours a day, every day for several years, even decades. However, because of the demand for non-extraction treatment, lip prominence, and reduction of "dark triangles," retention of the entire maxillary arch shape at night is often required [2].

Removable retainers

Traditional retainers for the entire maxillary arch, such as Hawley retainers and van der Linden retainers are still used for retention (Figure 9.1). As an alternative for these traditional removable retainers, invisible retainers (aligners) have been used successfully for several decades [3–5]. In the lower arch, the arch form will be normally maintained by the pressure equilibrium between the cheek and the tongue musculature. For custom orthodontic appliance systems, such as Insignia, the outline of the alveolar bone in the mandible (the mantrough) is visible during the virtual arch correction of the segmented teeth.

So it should be easy to maintain the lower cuspid distance during orthodontic treatment. Maintaining the distance between the lower cuspid distance could increase the stability of the lower arch after correction [6]. If removable appliances in the mandible are required, invisible retainers (passive aligners) can be the removable retainer of choice because of the inaccurate fit of most removable retainers with clasps. For patients with temporomandibular joint (TMJ) problems, gnathologic splints in the maxillary or mandibular arch designed in a virtual articulator and printed with three-dimensional (3D) printers can be used. If a cone beam computer tomography radiograph (CBCT) and a gnathologic registration (such as a SICAT registration) is available, a dental splint can then be designed on the CBCT/intraoral scan superimposition images and then printed in 3D.

Custom positioners, activators, and "Damon splints" can be used to maintain the interarch relation after orthodontic correction of class II or class III malocclusions. For patients with sleep apnea or who snore intensively, mandibular repositioning appliances (MRAs) could be useful after orthodontic treatment to reduce these problems, and these appliances will also retain the maxillary and mandibular arches. (Figure 9.2). Before prescription of an MRA, a medical checkup of these sleep

Digital Planning and Custom Orthodontic Treatment, First Edition. Edited by K. Hero Breuning and Chung H. Kau.
© 2017 John Wiley & Sons, Inc. Published 2017 by John Wiley & Sons, Inc.

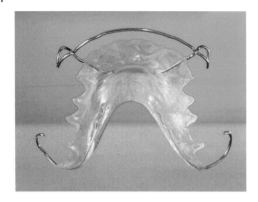

Figure 9.1 A Hawley removable retainer. Company: Ortholab.

problems by medical specialists is required. The workflow to make these appliances (impressions, design, and fabrication) can be traditional (an impression, lab order made by the orthodontist, and fabrication in the orthodontic lab), but a computer-aided design (CAD) and computer-aided manufacturing (CAM) workflow (intraoral scanning, design of the appliances in the lab, and fabrication of the appliances with 3D

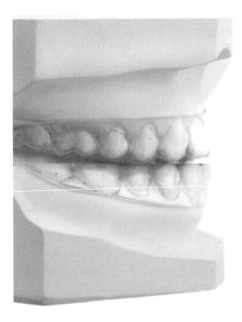

Figure 9.2 A mandibular repositioning appliance. Company: Ortholab.

printing machines) is becoming increasingly popular. Alternatively, the digital models can be printed and then the retainer appliances can be fabricated in the traditional way.

CAD/CAM retention wires

Permanent retention has now become the method of choice for stabilization of the incisors and cuspid region after orthodontic treatment. In an attempt to reduce the amount of fixed retainer failures and to increase the efficiency of the actual retention of the dentition by retainers, different materials for retainer fabrication and different methods to fabricate and position the retainers have been presented [7, 8]. An ideal fixed retainer should fit perfectly to each tooth selected. The retainer should prevent dental movement but should allow some physical movement. Cleaning of the tooth itself and the interproximal contacts should be easy. Removal of calculus by the dentist or the oral hygienist should be possible without the need to remove the retainer. The wire and the connection between the wire and the dentition should be sustainable. With the use of digital dental models made near the end of orthodontic treatment to fabricate retention wires with CAD/CAM techniques, it is now possible to design, fabricate, and transfer appropriate retainers to the dentition, and precise placement and effective retention of the tooth position during an extended period can be expected.

Retainer wires which have been designed with CAD techniques and fabricated with CAM techniques should be easy and accurately positioned and attached to the dentition [9]. This fabrication method to make retainers was developed by Dr. Pascal Schumacher from Germany. One of the companies offering this kind of retainer is Memotain. The production of this retention wire starts with a digital model of the patient. In a traditional workflow, an impression is used to make a plaster cast. This plaster model is then

Figure 9.3 Registration of the occlusion can be used to prevent failures.
Company: 3Shape.

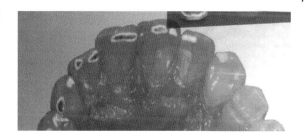

scanned with a desktop scanner to transfer the plaster model into a digital dental model. If an intraoral scanner is used to make an impression, the stereolithographic (STL) files of the scan can be used for digital model fabrication and will then be used to design a retainer wire according to the orthodontist's prescription.

For patients treated with lingual appliances, the brackets can then be virtually removed with software programs, such as Ortho-Analyser, to facilitate retainer design and to enable a digital design of the transfer tray. To prevent occlusal contacts between the maxillary retainer and the incisal edge of the lower incisors, the occlusal contacts between the upper and lower dentition are evaluated. In several software programs, such as Ortho-Analyser, it is possible to simulate lateral and frontal movements of the mandible in the virtual articulator. To prevent retainer wire failure the position of the upper wire retainer should be adapted to the location of the occlusal stops and functional contacts after evaluation of static and functional movements of the dentition in the virtual articulator (Figure 9.3).

Fabrication of the retainer wire

Computers and lasers will be used to cut the retainer out of a block of nitinol. According to the prescription the Memotain retainer, the dimensions of the retainer currently fabricated are 0.3 mm × 0.3 mm and this retainer wire is fabricated from a pseudo-elastic material. After the process of cutting the wire out of the nitinol block with a laser beam,

the retainer wire is electro-polished and finished (Figure 9.4). The flexibility of the nitinol retainer wire allows some physiologic movement of the teeth, and this will reduce breakage and bonding failures of the wire. A physical model (the original plaster model or a printed digital model) can be used for accurate transfer of the retainer to the dentition (Figure 9.5).

As an alternative, an indirect bonding jig can be designed in the Ortho-Analyser software and printed, without the need for a physical dental model.

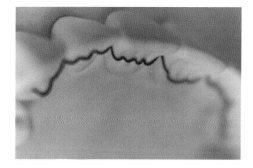

Figure 9.4 A custom-made retainer made from nitinol.
Company: Memotain.

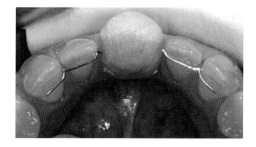

Figure 9.5 An indirect bonding jig made on a physical model.
Company: Memotain.

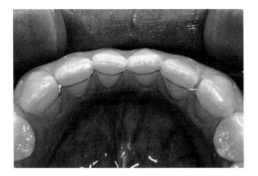

Figure 9.6 Optimal fit of the lingual retainer. Company: Memotain.

In a recent study, the accuracy of the computer-aided planning and the actual placement of the retainers were tested. The researchers concluded that: "Positional deviations were significantly less than 0.5 mm. They were very small in the horizontal and sagittal planes and moderately larger in the vertical plane" [9]. So highly precise intraoral results may be achieved by transferring 3D virtual setups for lingual retainers to the actual patients (Figure 9.6). This CAD/CAM strategy of making retainers can offer high predictability even in anatomically demanding regions and in the presence of limited space.

Advantages of these CAD/CAM retainers

This CAD/CAM process for orthodontic retention should result in the following advantages for the clinician:

- optimal fit of the retainer;
- optimal transfer of the retainer to the planned position on the dentition;
- increased comfort for the patient;
- less breakage of the wires (the wires are not bent);
- occlusal disturbances can be prevented;
- easy to clean (for the patient and the dentist);
- easy to be replaced if the wire is lost.

References

1 Littlewood, S.J., Millett, D.T., Doubleday, B., *et al.* (2016) Retention procedures for stabilising tooth position after treatment with orthodontic braces. *Cochrane Database Syst. Rev.*, **29** (1), CD002283.

2 Fleming, P.S., Dibiase, A.T., and Lee, R.T. (2008) Arch form and dimensional changes in orthodontics. *Prog. Orthod.*, **9** (2), 66–73.

3 Thickett, E. and Power, S. (2010) A randomized clinical trial of thermoplastic retainer wear. *Eur. J. Orthod.*, **32** (1), 1–5.

4 Mai, W., He, J., Meng, H., *et al.* (2014) Comparison of vacuum-formed and Hawley retainers: a systematic review. *Am. J. Orthod. Dentofacial Orthop.*, **145** (6), 720–727.

5 Kalha, A.S. (2014) Hawley or vacuum-formed retainers following orthodontic treatment? *Evid. Based Dent.*, **15** (4),110–111.

6 Yu, Y., Sun, J., Lai, W., *et al.* (2013) Interventions for managing relapse of the lower front teeth after orthodontic treatment. *Cochrane Database Syst. Rev.*, **6** (9), CD008734.

7 Renkema, A.M., Al-Assad, S., Bronkhorst, E., *et al.* (2008) Effectiveness of lingual retainers bonded to the canines in preventing mandibular incisor relapse. *Am. J. Orthod. Dentofacial Orthop.*, **134** (2), 179e1–8.

8 Renkema, A.M., Renkema, A., Bronkhorst, E., and Katsaros, C. (2011) Long-term effectiveness of canine-to-canine bonded flexible spiral wire lingual retainers. *Am. J. Orthod. Dentofacial Orthop.*, **139** (5), 614–621.

9 Wolf, M., Schumacher, P., Jäger, F., *et al.* (2015) Novel lingual retainer created using CAD/CAM technology: evaluation of its positioning accuracy. *J. Orofac. Orthop.*, **76**, 164–174.

10

The Invisalign System

Orhan Tuncay

Introduction

The Invisalign System is similar to a language: everyone uses it, but with notable differences. The differences could be in the accent, choice of words and slang, introduction of words from other languages, and the like. It is also in the voice and articulacy of the speaker and the eloquence and fluency of the writer. Interestingly, despite all such nuances, in the end, the goals of communication are attained in some form. The question remains, however: do goals affect the use of language just as language might shape the goal of the communication? The spirit of the above questions is seen in orthodontic treatment. Treatment goals vary from one practitioner to the next. The choices of appliances, too, vary as do the implementation of the chosen appliance. In the end, patients are treated to the satisfaction of the patient or the clinician, or both. But what determines satisfaction?

The Objective Grading System criteria offered by the American Board of Orthodontics cannot always represent or satisfy all the goals of appropriate treatment, especially in the adult patient. Issues such as the patient's quality of life, ease of treatment, pain of treatment, or length of treatment all matter. The orthodontist's measures of quality in occlusion, esthetics, ease of treatment, frequency of patient visits, treatment time, and the like also matter. It is not unreasonable to say the

unabridged ease of treatment is just as important as the alignment of teeth.

Arguably, elements of ease of treatment are the burden of treatment and perceived excellence of the result. These are defined collaboratively by the orthodontist and the patient. Concrete numerical tools of measure for these concepts, perhaps regretfully, do not exist for global applicability. The focus of this chapter, therefore, is to communicate a process, a flowchart, to deliver efficiency in treatment within the context of the patient's quality of life.

Predictable performance of aligners

Gingival response

The long-known fact that mechanics affect biology and biology affects mechanical performance will be the framework of this chapter. Whereas the mechanics of tooth movement is a rather limited field, biology of periodontal tissue is not that well understood and is a highly complex phenomenon. The predictable elements of periodontal soft tissue responses adhere to the realities of published research.

We discovered, a while back, that orthodontic movement of teeth is due to remodeling of periodontal tissues [1]. This

Digital Planning and Custom Orthodontic Treatment, First Edition. Edited by K. Hero Breuning and Chung H. Kau.
© 2017 John Wiley & Sons, Inc. Published 2017 by John Wiley & Sons, Inc.

remodeling response is an inflammatory reaction and akin to wound healing. It may be assumed the degree, duration, and magnitude of force application will determine how compliantly the tissues will remodel. Closure of a midline diastema provides the best illustration. With fixed appliances and elastic chains, one ends up with a Christmas ball decoration because of the high magnitude of forces applied by the elastic chain (Figure 10.1a). With aligners, however, forces are applied in a controlled manner and more gently. It results in a compliant gingival tissue remodeling response (Figure 10.1b, c).

Periodontal and dental health status

There is a plethora of reports in the literature on how teenage kids have difficulty in maintaining good oral hygiene, and resultant white spot lesions. A multicenter private practice-based study of Invisalign performance reported superior plaque and gingival indices, and an absence of white spot lesions (Figure 10.2a, b) [2].

Recently, however, the absence of white spot lesions is replaced by incisal carious lesion. Occasionally, teenagers will drink high-sugar beverages without removing the aligners. Consequently, the extended exposure of incisal edge enamel will turn carious (Figure 10.3).

Influence of adjacent teeth

Complete tracking of teeth in the aligner is critical to the performance of aligners. For predictable performance, tooth movement built-into the aligner must be fully exhausted before the patient moves on to the next aligner in the series. It is not uncommon that at least one tooth does not track well. In such instances, it is wise to not blame the non-tracking tooth but look at the adjacent teeth instead. Oftentimes, the non-tracking tooth is next to a long-rooted tooth. Long-rooted teeth do not move as readily as the adjacent teeth would like. All moving teeth require adjacent teeth to get out of their way (Figure 10.4).

In Figure 10.4, white areas on the central teeth indicate the aligner is still active and has plenty of energy left. Until all the built-in energy for the centrals is exhausted, there will be considerable space between the plastic and other tooth surfaces. Accordingly, the clinician would be wise to extend, in ClinCheck,

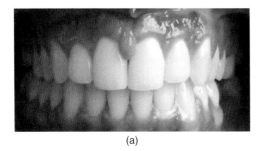

(a)

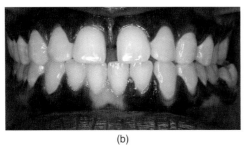

(b)

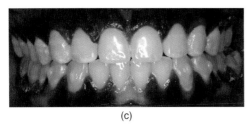

(c)

Figure 10.1 (a) In fixed appliance treatment the midline diastemas are most commonly closed with the aid of chain elastics. It may be presumed chain elastics pull too hard and too fast to create the red Christmas ball effect; (b) and (c) In contrast, aligner treatment with its programmed light force application allows remodeling of gingival tissues and prevents bunching.
Company: Align Technology, Inc.

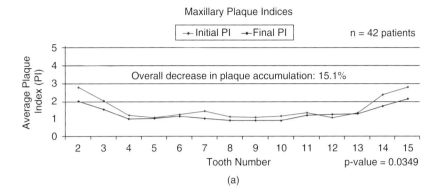

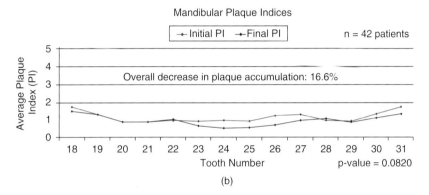

Figure 10.2 (a and b) Effects of aligner treatment on periodontal health and enamel white spot lesions are superior to what is seen in patients wearing fixed appliances. Source: [3]. Reproduced with permission of JCO.

such phases of treatment. Extended wear of aligners (e.g. by 3 or 4 weeks) is another option.

Another reason for poor tracking could be stiffness of the plastic. If there are too many attachments close to each other, all those bumps will stiffen the plastic. This is similar to how papers in a corrugated form make a stiff corrugated cardboard. The stiffened plastic, in turn, will have difficulty snapping on to the attachments and teeth. The ideal plastic is the one that is elastic and stretchable enough to snap on and push the teeth with its elasticity (Figure 10.5a, b).

Another common reason for lost tracking is inadequate number of hours clocked on the aligner. Too few hours of wear time will not exhaust the built-in energy and tooth

movement. And if the patient keeps changing aligners before the necessary hours are clocked, more crowding than existed before treatment will develop.

Unwanted tipping of teeth in extraction cases

A newly inserted aligner will house the space that the tooth or teeth will move to. It cannot be a plastic shrink-wrap around the tooth. If it were, tooth would have no place to move. That said, movement has to be controlled for the tooth to fill the space waiting for the tooth. It is the clinician's responsibility to design the force systems to "prevent" tipping. The design might incorporate special attachments, sequencing of tooth movements, adjustments of aligner stiffness, and

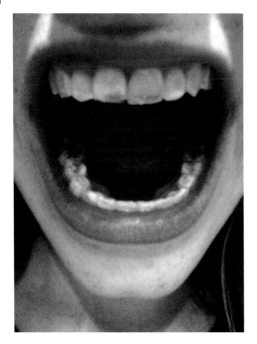

Figure 10.3 Incisal edge caries not seen until the introduction of aligner treatment, may be attributed to lack of brushing after consumption of sugar-laden beverages.
Company: Align Technology, Inc.

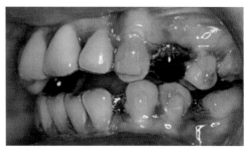

Figure 10.4 Pressure indicator paste discloses the aligner contact points.
Company: Align Technology, Inc.

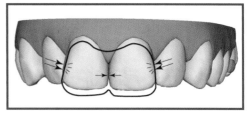

Figure 10.6 The ill-fitting aligner is more likely to create or compound a problem by applying pressure to unwanted areas of the teeth than do good.
Company: Align Technology, Inc.

the like. The essence of successful space closure lies in "prevention" of tipping.

Tipping may be prevented or minimized by allowing the plastic to surround the tooth in a cupping manner mesially, distally and buccolingually. Accordingly, the ClinCheck should be designed in such a manner that there is room is made on the mesial and distal surfaces. This statement infers separation of the tooth that requires prevention of tipping from the adjacent teeth. This strategy also applies to premolar extraction treatments (Figure 10.7a–c).

In premolar extraction treatments, it must be understood that as the anterior teeth are retracted the aligner length decreases. The

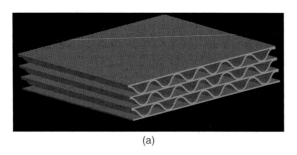

(a)

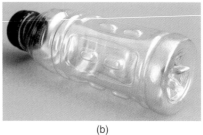

(b)

Figure 10.5 (a and b) The corrugation in paper or plastic stiffens the material.
Company: Align Technology, Inc.

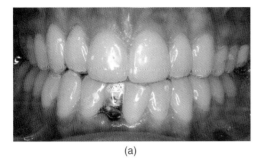

(a)

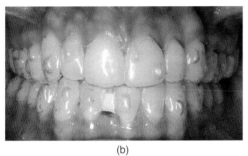

(b)

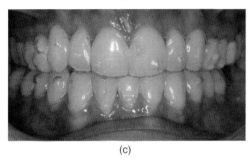

(c)

Figure 10.7 (a–c) Segmental mechanics to move the lateral tooth requires full "cupping" of the tooth with no distractions. In ClinCheck only one tooth should be moved at a time until space is closed and all roots are parallel.
Company: Align Technology, Inc.

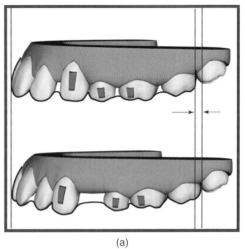

(a)

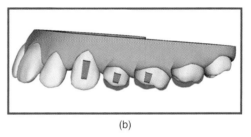

(b)

Figure 10.8 (a and b) In premolar extraction cases, as incisors are retracted the aligner length decreases. In turn, pressure is applied to the molars no different than a stretched rubber band; it pulls from both ends. In the absence of measures to prevent unwanted molar movements, these teeth tip uncontrollably.
Company: Align Technology, Inc.

decrease in length inevitably applies a force to push the molars mesially. This action is akin to a rubber band stretched from the anterior to the posterior teeth. The rubber band will pull from both ends. Accordingly, if the plan is to lock in and hold the molars steady, special precautions must be taken. If not, teeth will tip into the extraction space. Such tipping is more noticeable in the mandibular arch (Figure 10.8a and b).

In the event tipping is uncontrollable, segmental fixed appliances need to be employed as auxiliary appliances. Once the tipped teeth are uprighted, aligner treatment is reinstated to finish the treatment (Figure 10.9a–j).

Much of the tipping is due to the hourglass shape of periodontal ligament space. Thus, any magnitude, duration, or direction of force will be distributed within the periodontal ligament space such that the "hourglass" shape will promote a tipping movement more readily than bodily [2]. Accordingly, measures that overpower this tendency must be placed in the system (Figure 10.10a–h).

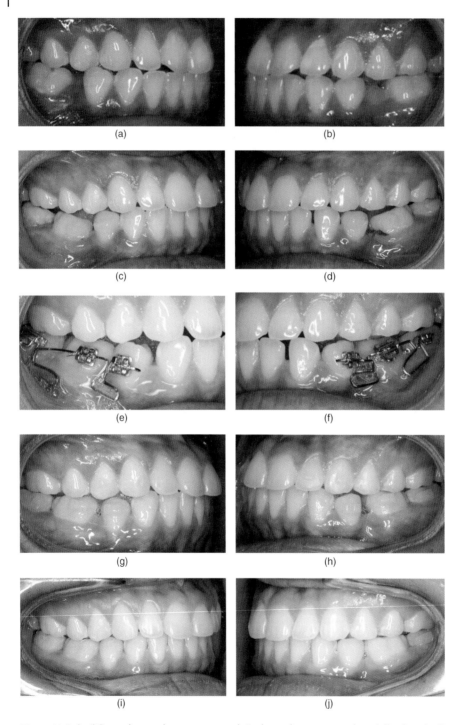

Figure 10.9 (a–j) Second premolars are extracted. As the molars are moved mesially, they tip. Root uprighting with segmental fixed appliances is necessary. Once the roots at the extraction site are parallel or overcorrected, treatment is finished with aligners.
Company: Align Technology, Inc.

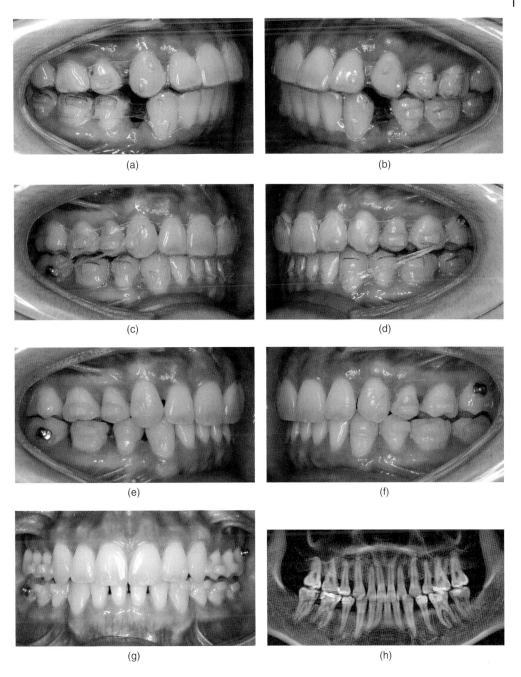

Figure 10.10 (a–h) In this four 1st premolar extraction case, long and prominent attachments are used to "prevent" tipping. Note the parallelism of the roots as the space is closed. The need for segmental fixed appliances to be parallel to the roots is removed.
Company: Align Technology, Inc.

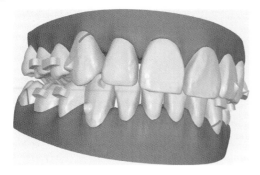

Figure 10.11 The prominent attachments simultaneously aid in extrusion and torqueing of the posterior teeth.
Company: Align Technology, Inc.

The old-fashioned rectangular attachments are best suited to this. These attachments must have dimensions that are: 5 mm long, 2 mm wide, and 1.5 mm prominent. The optimized attachments seen in the ClinCheck are clever designs for tooth movement but do not "prevent" undesirable tipping. At times, the aligner must have a strong grip on the tooth because the tooth shape is not favorable. Attachments serve to change the surface shape and characteristics of the tooth so that the aligner can snap on to the attachments for better grip. An aligner, after all, is a mere slipcover. It does not have the grip. The clinician must create the grip in the ClinCheck. If these aggressive attachments are used in large numbers, because they make the aligner plastic stiffer, molars can be locked in place, which will improve the prognosis (Figure 10.10a–h).

The prominent rectangular attachments also provide significant ability to create biomechanical "moments" and "couples" to torque teeth (Figure 10.11).

Extrusion of maxillary laterals

Anterior teeth extrude when retracted because the path of retraction creates an "arc" as the incisal edges move distally. It is commonly referred to as "relative extrusion."

If on the other hand, pure extrusion (along the long axis of the tooth) is required, challenges of movement and of retention can be frustratingly difficult. Pure extrusion of laterals with the aligners has never been easy. It could be due to: (1) adjacent teeth influences, (2) attachment design, or (3) periodontal ligament special fibers. These causes may be resolved by modifications to the appliance and duration of force application, thus overpowering the periodontal structures. The mechanical influence of adjacent teeth is discussed above. We will now give special attention to attachment design.

As stated above, if a tooth cannot engage the tooth as it needs to, the tooth shape must be changed to create handles for the plastic to grip. This change in surface morphology is facilitated by attachments. In pure extrusion, there is much soft tissue resistance that must be overcome. Currently, we don't know whether the beveled optimized attachments will always be particularly suited for this. Common clinical experience leads the clinician to choose intrusion of the posterior segments. But if the patient does not show any posterior vertical anomalies, pure extrusion is the only option to correct the open bite. Accordingly, if the attachment design is changed to a rectangular $5 \times 2 \times 1.5$ mm type then the plastic can find surfaces to snap on to and grip. Pure extrusion can be achieved with the aid of such attachment design (Figure 10.12a–k).

Resistance of soft tissues to remodeling is a principal obstacle in tooth movement [4]. The gingival tissues especially will either bunch up or simply won't remodel fast enough. In contrast, bone is the best friend the clinician ever had; it gets out of the way readily. For example, a tooth will erupt through the bone rapidly but then will get caught under the gingival tissue and take forever to erupt into the oral cavity.

It is important to note and to know that the root and periodontal ligament structures continue forming long after the crown

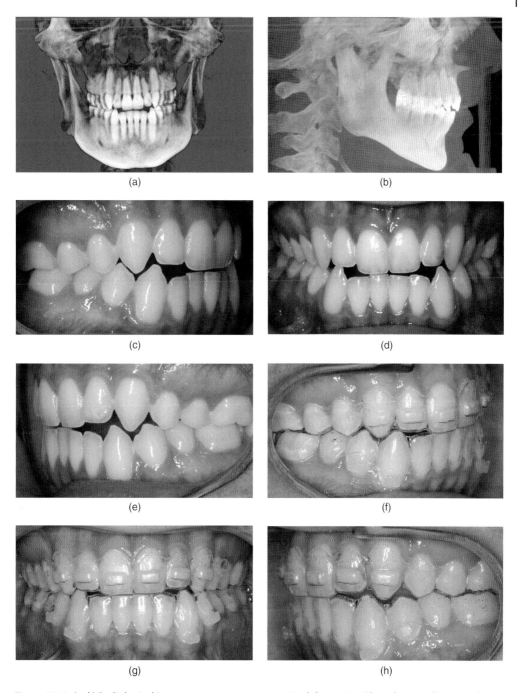

Figure 10.12 (a–k) Radiological images suggest no excess vertical dimension. Thus, the open bite must be corrected by pure extrusion of upper incisors. Long prominent rectangular attachments enable the aligner to snap on and pull the teeth with the aid of vertical elastics.
Company: Align Technology, Inc.

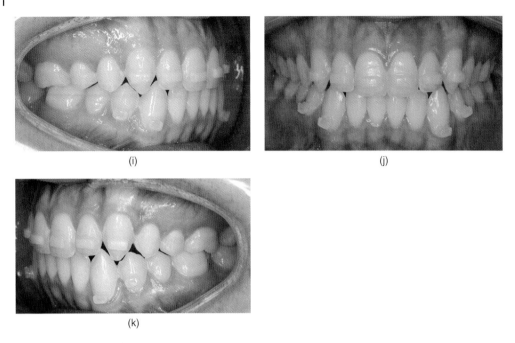

(i)

(j)

(k)

Figure 10.12 (*Continued*)

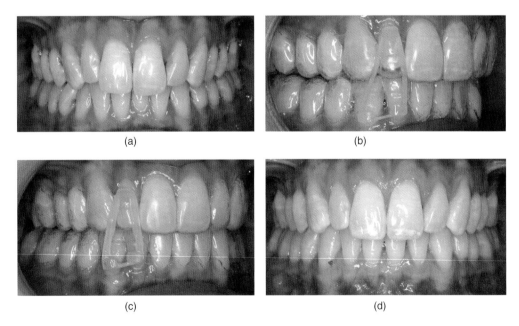

(a)

(b)

(c)

(d)

Figure 10.13 (a–d) Extrusion of maxillary laterals can be unpredictable. Certainly, retention can be disappointing. Fixed retention helps. In this case the right lateral did not erupt. Application of vertical elastics clearly helped, but subsequently the retention check came with a disappointment. Patient did not agree to a fixed retainer.
Company: Align Technology, Inc.

has become visible in the oral cavity. Most publications assume the composition of the periodontal ligament is uniform. But some define the periodontal ligaments by their location and orientation. We argue that, whereas the oblique orientation of the fibers defines their function to accommodate chewing type forces, the vertically oriented apical group of fibers adhere the root apex to the tooth socket. They are not designed to be stretched [4]. This characteristic makes extrusion a very difficult movement with the light forces of the aligner [5]. Fixed appliances overpower these fibers, but during the retention period the newly formed or remodeled fibers pull the tooth back into the original position (Figure 10.13a–d).

Developmental stages of the tooth and surrounding periodontal structures significantly affect the prognosis of extrusion. It may be argued that in the child patient these fibers have not yet formed, as the apex has not yet completed its development [3]. If there is no apical closure one may assume there are no apical fibers present. This postulate explains why adult teeth are more difficult to extrude and maintain. It should be noted, however, the argument applies to pure extrusion along the long axis of the tooth. Relative extrusion does not substantively involve the apical fibers. As the crowns are tipped, apices do not travel large distances.

In summary, to develop a more perfect predictability of tooth movement with the gentle forces of aligners, orthodontics must understand the biomechanical characteristics of the periodontal tissues. Treatment based on the genetic profile, metabolic state, vascular supply, and hydration levels of these collagenous tissues may be expected to remove much of the mystery.

References

1 Chumbley, A.B. and Tuncay, O.C. (1986) The effect of indomethacin (an aspirin-like drug) on the rate of orthodontic tooth movement. *Am. J. Orthod. Dentofac. Orthop.*, **869**, 312–314.

2 Mandel, U., Dalgaard, P., and Viidik, A. (1986) A biomechanical study of the human periodontal ligament. *J. Biomech.*, **19**, 637–645.

3 Tuncay, O.C., Bowman, S.J., Amy, B.D., and Nicozisis, J.L. (2013) Aligner treatment in the teenage patient. *JCO*, **2**, 115–119.

4 Tuncay, O.C. and Killiany, D.M. (1986) The effect of gingival fiberotomy on the rate of tooth movement. *Am. J. Orthod. Dentofac. Orthop.*, **89**, 212–215.

5 Tuncay, O.C. (ed.) (2006) Biologic elements of tooth movement, in *The Invisalign System*, Quintessence, Berlin.

11

Custom Lingual Appliances

Part 1: The History of Incognito

Neil Warshawsky

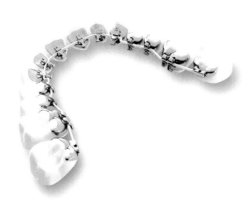

Back around the turn of the 21st century the orthodontic world was centered on plaster models and two-dimensional (2D) X-rays for diagnosis and diagnostic photographs to assist in treatment planning. At that point, the idea of digital photographs and models was still pretty new, the state of the art in equipment was digital 2D X-rays, and the clear aligner industry was in its infancy. In order to have esthetic orthodontic therapy your choices were either ceramic brackets, metal brackets in twin or self-ligation, or premade metal lingual brackets that utilized premade lingual wires. Custom orthodontics was not a reality. The best a practitioner could do was to utilize an indirect bonding tray to optimize bracket position to be more efficient. In short, the industry was not ready to go 100% custom at that point in time.

The new century did, however, bring some promise. There were some exciting ideas being developed at the time in Europe. A team of engineers formed a company named OraMetrix. They gathered across two continents in an effort to develop a multi-axis robot that could custom bend arch wires in three planes. By capturing three-dimensional (3D) data from teeth, the robot was able to create custom finishing bends in multiple wires and formats (i.e. copper nickel titanium (NiTi), stainless steel, TMA, Blue Elgiloy) to align the teeth. The key to this success was the ability to overcome poor bracket position. In effect, the bracket was just acting as a handle on the tooth. Gathering the 3D data proved to be the difficult part of the task. OraMetrix resolved their acquisition issues by developing one of the first commercially available chairside intraoral scanners. It created a 3D file and allowed them to create software to electronically segment teeth and establish a completely digital setup (DSL) or "target" of the teeth. The robot was then able to create compensating bends in the arch wires out of copper NiTi, TMA, and other materials to facilitate finishing orthodontic cases at a superior level. This custom arch wire was trade named suresmile. The wires fabricated by the suresmile system can be used with all types and brands of brackets.

Digital Planning and Custom Orthodontic Treatment, First Edition. Edited by K. Hero Breuning and Chung H. Kau.
© 2017 John Wiley & Sons, Inc. Published 2017 by John Wiley & Sons, Inc.

The robot's greatest strength was its ability to negate the bracket position, thus compensating for the position of the wire slot when less than ideal. The system, though, had its share of problems. It was expensive, as you had to purchase a separate network and install it in your office to communicate with OraMetrix. Their results showed that cases finished faster (almost 38%) as well as better. Although results of their effort were very promising, there was a glaring aspect still missing. The wires were 3D and the bends were oftentimes large and unsightly. In addition, the wires could be exceptionally active and proved difficult to place. The suresmile system was able to expedite quality of care for sure, but it was unable to do it in a cosmetic manner as the brackets were labial and visible. There was a void in the cosmetic orthodontic world and it clearly exposed the need to create a more cosmetic orthodontic bracket with the predictability of a robotic wire.

The answer came from an unlikely source. Dr. Dierck Wiechmann is an orthodontist who practices in Bad Essen, Germany. As an orthodontics graduate student, he investigated improving lingual orthodontics. His graduate study investigated using a robotic wire to predictably improve orthodontic efficiency. However, unlike the suresmile system, he felt that lingual orthodontics was the obvious choice for a cosmetic solution. To minimize the required number of bends, his team decided that it would be more efficient to reverse engineer the case. His funds were limited and certainly he did not have the venture capital or the access to the items that OraMetrix had. His system was more "analog," as it required high-quality PVS impressions to pour custom models of the case. A custom wax setup of the malocclusion was created by hand to ideally create a physical target of the final occlusal position. Commercially available lingual orthodontic brackets were then set on the wax setup model to create a flat wire plane (based on the TARG

system) to build to. Once the flat wire plane was designed, the setup would be scanned and a simpler two-axis robot would be used to pre-bend all of the working arch wires for the practitioner to treat out the case. Dr. Wiechmann's master thesis proved to be an excellent alternative at the time, as it demonstrated an efficient way to orthodontically treat teeth in a truly cosmetic fashion. Once he was done with his studies, Top-Service orthodontic labs were formed. He was determined to change the orthodontic world.

Operating out of Bad Essen did not prove to be a limiting factor. However, the premade orthodontic brackets the lab was utilizing did. In an effort to seek out a better solution, the lab set out to create a better custom lingual bracket. Custom 3D wax printing proved to be the media they would use to create the brackets. At first the brackets were almost exact copies of the bracket they initially started with (Ormco 7th Generation Lingual). But the problem still existed that the bracket body was so large it would interfere on deep bite cases with creating the final incisal guidance. It was just a matter of time before the proper design came. Eventually, it was determined that, to get the bracket closer to the tooth, the wire plane needed to be tipped 90 degrees rotating the wire plane. Instead of an edgewise system, a ribbon arch would be chosen for the next generation lingual. Trade named Incognito, it set out to deliver, as the name implied, completely invisible custom lingual solutions. The system grew in popularity in Europe and by 2005 it was the most popular custom lingual bracket system sold. The ribbon arch proved to be an exciting development. With time, the addition of custom auxiliaries such as saddle bands that did not separate teeth interproximally, custom Class II correction utilizing both Herbst and Forsus[TM] applications, light cured indirect Clear Precision Trays[TM] (CPT), a multilingual customer support team, and several European schools recognizing and teaching the Incognito system, this lingual platform was gaining popularity. Worldwide, though, it was very limited in its distribution. It lacked a strong presence outside of Europe and was unable to gain worldwide acceptance without a global sales team dedicated to client service and development.

Well, that all soon changed as the American Branch of Incognito, which was managed by Ruedger Rubbert and Lea Ellermeier Nesbit, was purchased in 2007 by 3M. As the large corporate entity wrapped its arms around this small boutique company, it was clear that, in order to succeed in incorporating this new brand into their oral care portfolio, they would need to further their reach with their investment to incorporate the European community where the product was met with much wider acceptance. The acquisition of the European branch, which included the Top-Service which was overseen personally by Wiechmann, was completed before the conclusion of 2008. The second purchase helped to establish a global presence for 3M with Incognito in over 70+ countries. This presence included sales and distribution channels in each of these countries, a multilingual live customer care support network, and a multifactorial teaching system where 3M would utilize the web, university programs, live hands-on programs, and study-club formats to educate users and elevate their skillset with regards to Incognito. For 3M this was the key to propelling Incognito forward and increase its acceptance worldwide.

3M recognized from the onset that they needed to make several key changes if they were going to gain global acceptance in the orthodontic community. They formed a global advisory committee of orthodontists, administrators, and research and development personnel from across the globe to come together to create a unified voice to help steer the product development. Meeting 1–2 times per year gave 3M the ability to discuss, design, clinically evaluate, and ultimately roll

out upgrades and improvements to Incognito. What became apparent in the process is that Incognito is in fact an elite system. It required its own certification and training course, and given where you lived in the world its delivery may be live or via the Internet. However, certification was not enough on its own to gain experience to be successful with such a novel system. Further training by both the orthodontists and the support staff would be required to become adept at this unique approach to orthodontic care. So as many people learn in many different ways and languages, it was evident that this system required multiple channels of continuing education: printed, online, and live customer care in several languages were all required to support such a comprehensive and unique system. Study clubs, users meetings, customized special instruments, and specialty adhesive would also be required to support what ultimately morphed into its own system. Given the magnitude and complexity of the requirements to support a system as complex as this, it is no wonder that a company such as 3M would be the ultimate owner necessary to propel this system to global acceptance. It's capability to treat any malocclusion while showing minimal hardware gave the term "hidden braces" a new meaning. It simply is, in this author's estimation, the finest, most complete orthodontic appliance system commercially available to date worldwide.

The reality of Incognito is that it is able to be customized to any individual's needs. Custom-built appliances we know fit better, work quicker, and hurt less. It has the capacity, given that it is custom made, to achieve sometimes near-impossible results when compared with any other orthodontic system available today. The process owes its success in large part to the fact that 3M recognized from the onset that with mass customization of any custom medical or dental product the design would need to be done in a systematic digital format with a series of checks and balances. The system today

Full
Digital
Workflow
precise
Treatment
Results

1. 3M™ True Definition scanner to capture the dentition

2. Unitek™ Treatment Management Portal to produce Digital setups

3. Digital Setup Lab

4. Unitek™ Treatment Management Portal to evaluate and approve setups in 3D

5. Computer-Aided Bracket design

6. Bracket manufacturing

7. Incognito™ Clear Precision Tray

8. Archwire Bending

9. Quality Assurance and Shipping

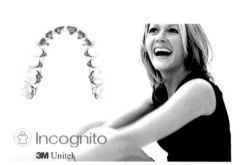

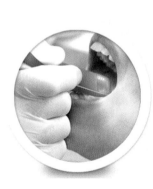

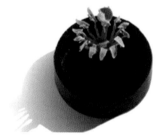

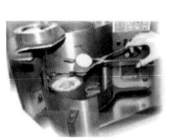

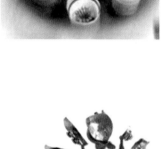

involves the most current technology available in dentistry, and is referred to as the "digital workflow." Although not all customers are currently utilizing all steps of the digital workflow at the moment, it is clear that the goal is for all cases to ultimately be built in this manner. This process is more accurate than the conventional lab process as it utilizes digital models for all planning and setup models. Since there are no stone models in this process, the process is inherently more accurate. All physical dental models, regardless of which material they are made of, will have shrinkage and porosity factors to contend with. Separating the individual stone teeth to reset them in wax to create an ideal occlusal setup is a very subjective process. Many errors can be associated with this process, whether desired or not. Again, in a digital workflow, this is not a factor, as the teeth can be electronically separated with no loss to the width of the teeth. So the real issue here is that a digital model of the patient must be created in order to initiate the digital workflow.

It is important to understand that any custom orthodontic appliance system, and not just Incognito, has a lot to benefit from being created entirely from a digital file. This new process of manufacturing via software is a "digital disruption." This "all digital" process standardizes the product for manufacturing. You do not have to worry about whether the impressions were poured and trimmed properly, if teeth were adequately sectioned for the manual waxup, or if UPS or FedEx lost your shipment. The digital disruption completely removed these steps from the equation by creating a new "electronic process" which ultimately is faster and more accurate.

Amongst the different regions of the world, certain subjective decisions may be applied to the subset of patients from that region. For example, in Asia there is a high percentage of extraction in the patient population. As a result the norms for these setups may be adjusted so that additional crown torque may be applied to this subset of patients.

A DSL made from stereolithographic (STL) files will be the most accurate. It is well known that PVS material has some degree of error. With Incognito's slot precision, it is critical to minimize *any* chance of error. Therefore, 3M is working hard to make Incognito a 100% digitally built system worldwide. It will not only that ensure the product is the most accurate it can be but also ultimately create a product delivered to the consumer faster, with fewer issues. Most importantly, if it can be digitally built, it has the promise to reduce cost to the consumer, as the entire manufacturing can be reduced by up to two weeks,

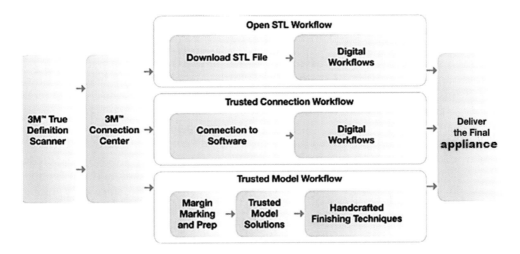

Digital

Manual

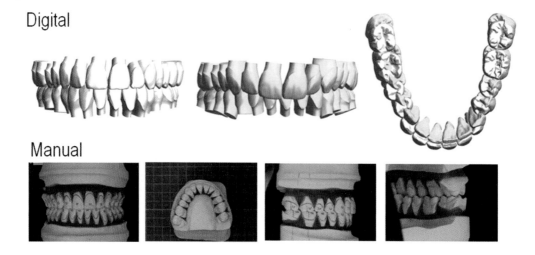

since it will not require FedEx or UPS to send PVS impressions into a 3M facility, it will not have to go through a sterilizing process once it is received, and it will not require two sets of impressions to be poured and quality controlled upon arrival at the manufacturing plant.

Initially, 3M cannot expect that all users worldwide will be able to obtain a digital impression of their patient. So in the event that the orthodontist uses PVS to impress their patient's teeth, 3M will start their foray into the digital workflow by pouring two sets of models from the PVS impressions. Once the models pass through quality control, they are mounted on an articulator, the teeth are sectioned apart by hand, and then an ideal as possible occlusion is created by setting the teeth in wax. The waxups are based on Dr. Larry Andrews' six keys of occlusion. Although this goal is not achieved in a majority of cases, it was and still seems to be a good place to start. Three-dimensional scanning of the waxups of the setups created in the lab was Incognito's answer to creating a digital manufacturing process. Although there was still the potential for error from physical models being poured, the teeth being cut apart and sectioned for setup, and the scanner not being properly calibrated, it was still

decided that this process had the potential for greater accuracy than any manual system.

It is this drive to create custom lab work which is fueling the next big game changer in orthodontics: digital impressions. Intraoral scanners have recently come to the technology forefront in dentistry as the new holy grail, with the promise to eliminate the dreaded physical impression. Just as vinyl LP albums, cassette tapes, and compact discs have blazed the trail for digital download or streaming of music, if successfully adopted digital impressions are sure to be the next industry trend. Of course, at the end of the day, it will only be adopted if orthodontists can make money and dentistry can be made easier, faster, and more precise. 3M is a global manufacturer of a kaleidoscope of dental products including, but not limited to, orthodontic bands and brackets, a host of dental materials for various types of tooth restorations, custom impression materials, and dental hand instrumentation to name a few. They recognized the overall need in dentistry for a relatively easy-to-use digital impression system. It was a critical development for them to achieve since a key product that they produced is impression material. Digital impressions were a reality as well as a "digital disruptor," and in order to compete in an all-digital world, they needed to be able to have an entry to compete with other digital systems that were simultaneously being developed. To answer the need for a digital yet economical solution to physical impression materials, 3M^{TM} created the True Definition Scanner to acquire digital intraoral impressions for dentistry in general. Their idea was that one scanner could be utilized regardless of what the desired manufacturing goal was. To be clear, the Trudef, as it is called, works on both a single tooth as well as an entire dental arch. It incorporates digital treatment planning and design, collaborating across multiple industry platforms regardless of brand. Most importantly, it reduces the time required to manufacture custom-made appliances.

This new process of appliance manufacturing, known as the digital workflow, surely has the potential to affect not just orthodontics but all parts of dentistry. For our purposes, this discussion will focus on how to use the 3M True Definition scanner to design and build custom Incognito lingual braces. Note that the digital workflow for construction of Incognito braces is not limited to the True Definition scanner from 3M. Both the second-generation iTero and the 3Shape Trios scanners are also currently accepted.

What must be remembered about the digital workflow is that success is not limited to the Incognito system. Once upon a time, digital X-rays were considered fancy equipment that few practices could utilize. Today they are considered the standard in dentistry. Digital impressions are sure to go in the same direction. The limiting factor today is hardware and its development, but this field is sure to improve over the coming years. Therefore, if you are unable to acquire a digital impression, today the lab will create an analog 3D scan on a benchtop scanner of a model that was poured from the impression you sent in. Once this extra step has been performed, the rest of the process from design to production of the Incognito appliance is the same.

Innovative Design for a Better Overall Experience

The 3M™ True Definition Scanner has the smallest wand on the market for fast and easy scanning. The lightweight wand is ergonomically balanced and allows one-handed scanning from multiple positions.

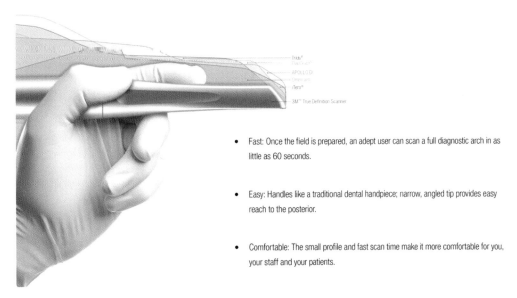

- Fast: Once the field is prepared, an adept user can scan a full diagnostic arch in as little as 60 seconds.

- Easy: Handles like a traditional dental handpiece; narrow, angled tip provides easy reach to the posterior.

- Comfortable: The small profile and fast scan time make it more comfortable for you, your staff and your patients.

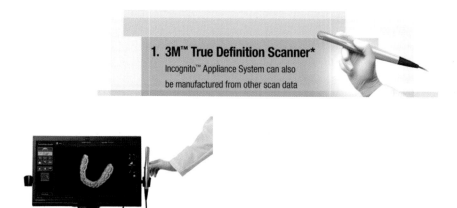

1. **3M™ True Definition Scanner***

Incognito™ Appliance System can also be manufactured from other scan data

The second step in the digital workflow following data acquisition is to access the Treatment Management Portal (TMP) to order your patient's Incognito case. There are a few parts of the world that still require paper order forms for new Incognito orders, but the intention is for all users with time to be able to go online to order custom appliances for their patients.

To begin your digital order you are required to have the TMP on your computer. TMP is free to users once they have completed a certification course. Currently, the program is not web-based and requires a PC to be downloaded for your use. It will not run on an iPAD or other mobile device as it is a rather robust program. Once the patient's basic details (birthdate, office location, ID number) are inputted, your order process can begin.

As a new patient in TMP you may request two different products from the platform. Either digital models or Incognito appliances. When ordering Incognito, you will automatically receive the initial malocclusion digital models on ABO style bases. This allows you to objectively compare the proposed DSL for Incognito to your initial malocclusion.

There are many diagnostic tools within TMP that you may utilize to confirm that the setup is what you are looking for. In addition, if you use Dolphin Imaging you have the option to upload your diagnostic information onto TMP so that all your tools will be in a single location for treatment planning purposes. Customer care will be able to visualize these records as well in the event that they need to confirm that the proposed treated plan meets your targeted treatment goal.

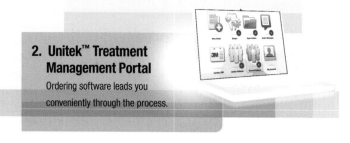

2. **Unitek™ Treatment Management Portal**

Ordering software leads you conveniently through the process.

Unitek™ Treatment Management Portal

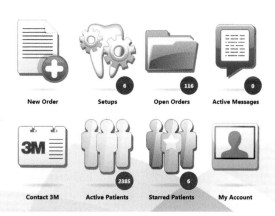

If you choose to use a digital impression as opposed to PVS material, you will automatically be taken to a dropdown menu of all digital impressions from your scanner that have been directed to 3M. You should find your patient in this box. Highlighting the patient will bring up a mini pictorial of the teeth. If the teeth in the image appear to be correct, you will then have the option to attach the scan to the manufacturing order. For this digital workflow there is nothing else to do to attach the scan to the order. The one thing that must be understood, though, is that, depending on which scanner you use, you will need to tell the scanner "where" to send the

images. It is not a very challenging process and once this has been done two or three times I am sure your team will get this process down.

Currently, there are three intraoral scanners that 3M has approved for manufacturing. They are the True Definition Scanner from 3M, the iTero scanner from Cadent, and the Trios scanner from 3Shape. As it currently stands, the 3M scanner is the lightest, the smallest, most accurate, and ironically the cheapest scanner available in the United States. This technology is sure to improve with time, but what must be understood is that it has a limited lifespan. Given what is

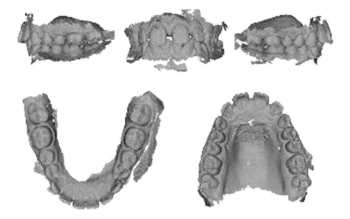

currently available, you can come to your own decision as to whether you are ready to purchase one.

Once the impression medium is chosen and attached, the order process begins. The first page contains all of the information regarding the order. The first few windows are by far the most important and must be paid close attention to. Arches to be treated must be chosen. You will have the opportunity in a single arch of treatment to set up the opposing arch. You will be able to dictate whether it is anterior only or comprehensive care. In the appliance section you will need to choose which product your patient needs: comprehensive or limited. In comprehensive you will need to choose how many teeth will be involved in movement. Your options are 4 to 4, 5 to 5, 6 to 6, or 7 to 7. Prices will automatically adjust with each option. Implants, bridges, and ankylosed teeth need to be marked so that they are not moved in the DSL setup. If the limited or LITE setup is chosen, only the anterior 6 teeth may move. This option will allow you to choose four wires (comprehensive comes with five wires). You may purchase up to eight brackets, and can even add splints between the premolars to prevent the posterior teeth from moving, but only the front six teeth move. Therefore, this product by default is my choice for minor relapse when I do not want to use an aligner system for correction. Lastly, in the lower third on the left side of the order screen a pictorial typically will "gray out" teeth that are not moving. You may mark extraction as well

as missing teeth as well as those mentioned above.

Next come treatment goals and objectives. This information is all being used to create your target setup, so be as descriptive as you can. The more information the designer has, the greater your likelihood to achieve an optimal setup. If diagnostic records have been uploaded, they will be visible at this point.

The second page is where you will order the physical braces. Again, you will only be able to order what you need based on the prescription you entered on the first page. There are endless combinations for comprehensive care. One clever part of this ordering tool is it will give you a representative diagrammatic picture of what you are ordering. Incognito is a uniquely different system than anything on the labial. It offers many custom features such as a ribbon arch wire, half occlusal pads, custom saddle bands that require no separation, easy entry terminal tubes, a lower self-ligation slot on the lower 6 anterior teeth, and many different types of anchorage. Herbst and Forsus attachments are available on the labial, as well as labial attachments on the buccal of bands. To customize a tooth is quite simple. Active teeth tend be gold colored on screen. The system will automatically populate the screen based on your order from page 1.

As an example, if you order "Lite" 3 = 3 you will have 6 teeth available to look at. The image prepopulates with a pictorial of what you are asking for, but you may make changes, like bracket vs tube and hook vs no hook on

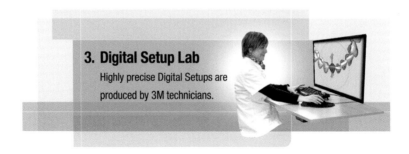

3. Digital Setup Lab

Highly precise Digital Setups are produced by 3M technicians.

a posterior tooth. To further customize or change something on a tooth, highlight the tooth in question and it will turn from gold to purple on screen. Once you do this look at the bottom of the page and you will see two lines of information. One line has to do with bracket vs. tube. The second line has to do with band vs bracket. Each has myriad choices including, but not limited to, half occlusal pads to open the bite.

At the top of page two in TMP there is a significant development that is now offered known as a CPT.

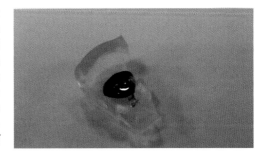

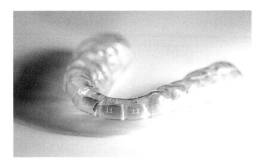

The CPT is an option in any case. It is an indirect bonding tray that is built directly from digital data. It has a soft silicone inner layer with a hard outer shell. The soft tray may be sectioned after the initial bonding appointment and it may be used as a rebonding jig to verify that if you need to rebond a bracket it will be bonded in the correct position for sure. It also allows the user to leverage other 3M strengths, and utilize RelyX

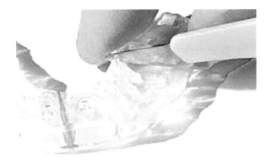

luting cement to bond the incognito to the teeth. RelyX is a dual-cured filled resin cement that contains a metal primer so there is no preparation of the gold bracket bases required to bond them. This simplifies the bonding process for incognito and it allows you to initially light cure the bonding tray. Previous to the CPT, I would have recommended the use of the putty tray but after extensive testing of the CPT, I do feel that this is the bonding tray of choice to attach the brackets. In any event if you are unclear how to use the ordering wizard to build the physical brackets and bands, there is a box at the bottom of page 2, where you may write in any requests with regards to the appliance design.

The third page of the ordering wizard concerns your wires. Toward the top of the page are some templates for extraction and non-extraction cases. You may quickly choose these and/or modify them to save time or you may create your own and save them if you so desire. The NiTi wires are automatically super elastic wires. You may opt for the gold-colored copper NiTi as well by checking the box at the bottom of the page. The wires have the option to have straight posterior segments in the event that you need to retract or distalize teeth. Your initial NiTi wire will be very flexible, and you will receive a spare in case it breaks. I usually suggest ordering the copper NiTi if your case exhibits crowding. I recommend the silver super elastic NiTi if you are starting with straight or relatively spaced teeth.

Archwire Selection (Archwire Selection Guide)

Archwire Material and Size	Upper Arch				Lower Arch			
	Extraction Straight Lateral Section	Straight Lateral Section Q1	Q2	Non-Extraction Individual Lateral Section	Extraction Straight Lateral Section	Straight Lateral Section Q3	Q4	Non-Extraction Individual Lateral Section
SE Ni-Ti								
0.012" round	▼	☐	☐	▼	▼	☐	☐	▼
0.014" round	▼	☐	☐	▼	▼	☐	☐	(1) ▼
0.016" round	(1) ▼	☐	☐	▼	▼	☐	☐	▼
0.018" round	▼	☐	☐	▼	▼	☐	☐	▼
0.016" x 0.022"	(1) ▼	☐	☐	▼	▼	☐	☐	(1) ▼
0.017" x 0.025"	▼	☐	☐	▼	▼	☐	☐	▼
0.018" x 0.025"	(1) ▼	☐	☐	▼	▼	☐	☐	(1) ▼
Steel								
0.016" round	▼	☐	☐	▼	▼	☐	☐	▼
0.018" round	▼	☐	☐	▼	▼	☐	☐	▼
0.016" x 0.022"	▼	☐	☐	▼	▼	☐	☐	▼
0.016" x 0.022" ET	▼	☐	☐	▼				
0.016" x 0.024"	▼	☐	☐	▼	▼	☐	☐	(1) ▼
0.016" x 0.024" ET	(1) ▼	☐	☐	▼				
0.018" x 0.025"	▼	☐	☐	▼	▼	☐	☐	▼
Beta III Titanium								
0.0175" x 0.0175"				▼				▼
0.0182" x 0.0182"				▼				▼
0.017" x 0.025"				(1) ▼				(1) ▼
0.0182" x 0.025"				▼				▼

Upper Wires Selected: 0   **Lower Wires Selected: 0**

One should remember that when utilizing the Incognito system in a case with crowding, you should not engage every tooth on the wire. I do recommend using stops to advance the wire and make space for the first visit or two. In the lower arch you may just engage the wire in the self-ligation slot and then eventually swing the wire into the slot. My personal protocol preferences automatically build a mild amount of expansion into all of my digital setups. This allows me to advance wires safely into the crowded cases. Brackets may be added as space is available but the key to success in this system is to tie the wire down tightly. If I could give one piece of advice it would be to tie the wires in as snugly as possible using a minimum of double overties on all of the anterior teeth. Power ties work even better to help to upright the

roots of the teeth. After a few months, place them in steel ligature "double overties." The Incognito system is an "en masse" retraction system. You must gather up all spaces from canine to canine and then retract your anterior teeth "en masse" to close extraction sites. When gathering space between the anterior teeth you will need to pull them together, even if the wire is a nitinol-based wire. Tying the teeth down tightly will upright the teeth so that you may get the full size steel wire 016 × 024 steel wire in for space closure. Remember it is a ribbon arch and not an edgewise system. Therefore steel ties should be on all brackets when retracting space. If you try to close spaces on anything but this steel wire you will encounter major problems with the alignment of the teeth. You must also use the double cable mechanics technique

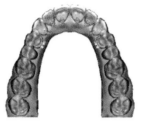
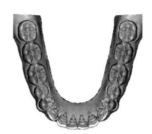

to retract the teeth or you are bound to experience what is referred to as the "bowing effect." When you are treating a case with extractions you have the option to order extra torque on the anterior teeth in your steel closing wire (referred to as .016″ × .024″ stainless steel in the Incognito system). It just helps to maintain incisor position when you are wearing elastics. It will not over-torque the teeth. It will just prevent the teeth from "dumping inward" as you retract extraction sites closed. To facilitate space closure you need to order straight segments on the posterior when retracting the teeth. You may add back your second order bends in your finishing wire, which typically is TMA by choice. Once your wires selection is complete, you will just need to sign your prescription in TMP and the manufacturing of your system will begin.

The setup for Incognito will be mostly, if not entirely, completed digitally by the time this book comes to print. Your setup instructions from your order will be followed, and after a few days inside the home menu of TMP you will receive a notice, and by email, that a setup is ready for review.

Within a week of the order being completed, work will begin to create your DSL, otherwise referred to as the DSL. When delivered, it will come with a list of instructions known as macros. The macros specifically discuss how the designer addressed the midline, arch form, molar classification, what tooth or teeth the setup is referenced around, the occlusal plane, and lastly any unique or specific instruction. Upon delivery your setup is available in TMP so you can critically view and evaluate it. There are many useful tools to help evaluate whether the setup is even possible let alone correct in terms of alignment. The model is a 3D active model, and so can be rotated and viewed from all angles inside the TMP software. However, I would recommend several of my favorite tools specifically when evaluating your models. The first thing that I turn on when evaluating my DSL is the blue overlay tool. Using a variable translucent lever, you can get a very accurate view of how much the teeth are moved in the setup. It is important to use this tool first, because it is possible from time to time that you may make an error in your

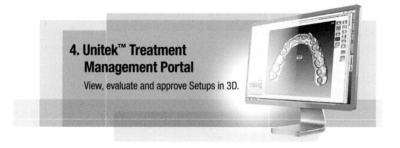

4. Unitek™ Treatment Management Portal
View, evaluate and approve Setups in 3D.

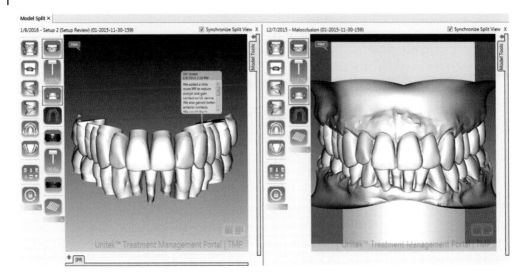

order. An example of this may happen when a molar is missing for an extended period. It may be obvious to you that the site will get an implant ultimately. However, if the tooth is missing and you have a protocol that says to close excess space unless told otherwise, the lab may close up all of the space because you forgot to tell it otherwise. The translucency tool is excellent for large global evaluations.

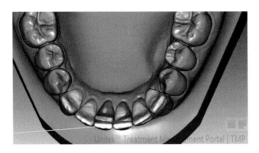

The next tool to use is a tool that locks the rotation of the DSL model to the initial malocclusion. It allows you to evaluate both models simultaneously. Again, it's a useful tool

to make sure the lab is designing what your patient requires and is capable of achieving.

When looking at symmetry one of the easiest tools to use is a transparent grid, which can be placed over the model axially, coronally, or sagittally. Since it is transparent, it is very easy to evaluate the arch form, smile design, and the amount of buccal width built into each case. There is a table at the base of the DSL that may be collapsed which contains a detailed IPR (interproximal reduction) chart. It discusses the extent and the location of the interproximal reduction.

Once reviewed, the last thing you need to pay attention to is at the bottom of the macros in the toolbox. Upon completion of your review of the DSL, you will have the option to either request a change and deny the model or accept it and initiate fabrication. To abandon a model and start afresh, click the "create new note box" above the macros ledger in the tools box. Then go to the DSL model and click on the area where you are dissatisfied. A note box will open up above

IPR	UR8	UR7	UR6	UR5	UR4	UR3	UR2	UR1	UL1	UL2	UL3	UL4	UL5	UL6	UL7	UL8	
UR					0.3 0.2	0.3 0.2	0.2 0.3	0.2	0.2 0.3 0.2	0.2 0.3 0.2 0.3							UL
	D M	D M	D M	D M	D M	D M	D M	M D	M D	M D	M D	M D	M D	M D			
LR																	LL
	LR8	LR7	LR6	LR5	LR4	LR3	LR2	LR1	LL1	LL2	LL3	LL4	LL5	LL6	LL7	LL8	

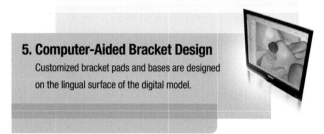

5. Computer-Aided Bracket Design

Customized bracket pads and bases are designed on the lingual surface of the digital model.

the macro box as well as on the DSL model. In here you need to type what you are dissatisfied with regarding the occlusion. You need to describe how you want to see it resolved. It is a clever way of indicating exactly what you do not like in the setup. There is no limit to the number of notes that you may create, *but* there is a limit to two revisions per setup. Anything beyond that will require an additional fee. Therefore you need to be explicit to get the result you are looking for. The final DSL model may be acknowledged by clicking on the "accept" button underneath the macro table and the case will automatically be placed into the queue for manufacturing.

Computer-aided bracket design starts by the creation of the custom bracket pads for every tooth that will receive a bracket. Once the pads are traced, bracket bodies are chosen based on the order in TMP. Each individual bracket will be customized based on the prescription in TMP. Bracket bodies are chosen from a custom library of bodies and then ligation hooks are tipped in and out of the plane so that they mimic the contour of the tooth surface. Because all brackets are customized, they can overcome most anatomical limitations.

The final step in the design stage is to transfer the custom-designed brackets from the DSL model back to the original malocclusion. Final trimming of the bracket pads will be done at this stage to ensure that there are no interferences between the brackets. Upon

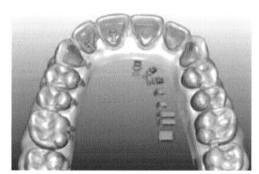

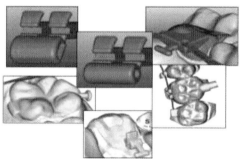

6. Bracket Manufacturing

The brackets are precision made in dental gold. Using a multi-step process.

7. Incognito™ Clear Precision Tray
This highly precise bonding tray is produced directly from digital data eliminating manual steps.

completion the brackets will start an extensive manufacturing process where they will be cast in dental gold, tumbled post casting, and polished to a high shine for intraoral placement. The process takes over 60 hours to complete including the fabrication of the indirect bonding CPT. Since transferring the bracket back to a physical model is a manual process with traditional indirect bonding, it adds the potential for error in placement of the brackets. This is why current thinking suggests bonding incognito brackets at the initial appointment with a custom precision tray.

This step will insure accuracy in the transfer as the tray is fabricated directly from digital data. It is composed of a soft clear silicone inner layer and a hard outer plastic layer. Brackets are individually placed into the soft clear tray based on the digital data. There is no special preparation required to be done to the back of the brackets as this protocol utilizes RelyX Luting cement to place the brackets on the teeth. This adhesive contains multiple primers for gold, non-precious metal, and plastic, and so no further special prepping will be required for the Incognito if this protocol is followed.

The last step for producing a reproducible product is to standardize the wires so that ideal arch form can be used in all wire formats from the initial leveling and aligning, up through the final detailing of the teeth. All wires are built on a robot, to ensure that the "ideal arch form" is used at every stage of the case.

Wires are available in multiple dimensions in each of the following materials: super elastic NiTi, copper NiTi, stainless steel, and TMA to finish. This approach prevents the round tripping of teeth. To incorporate extraction cases straight posterior segments are available to work the cases. In addition, intermediate arch forms are available where the distance between the cuspid offset may be adjusted to compensate for excessive crowding or spacing. Put simply, the range of choices is such that just about any configuration is possible. The wires once bent are taped to a 1:1 printed rendition of the final arch form.

The Incognito appliance system incorporates many features to facilitate alignment of the teeth. Owing to its many unique features, such as it is placed lingually—the wires area ribbon arch not an edgewise system, and

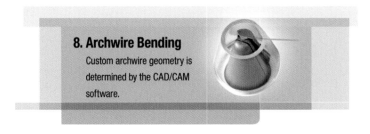

8. Archwire Bending
Custom archwire geometry is determined by the CAD/CAM software.

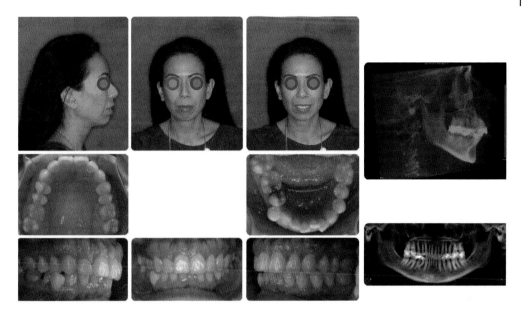

the digital workflow to reverse engineer the case—it is truly a unique mechanical concept. Let's review a case to help understand how it performs.

A 40.8-year-old Caucasian female presented to our office post treatment for some minor temporomandibular dysfunction. She had a nighttime full occlusal guard to prevent her from grinding her teeth. The patient was very specific about her desires and did not want to have any teeth extracted, nor would she consider any labial appliances for her orthodontic correction. She chose to use the Incognito appliance to correct and align her teeth. She presented with the following malocclusion:

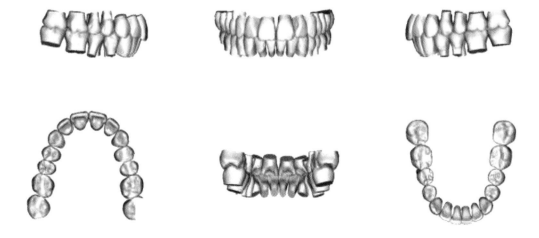

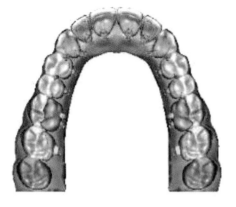
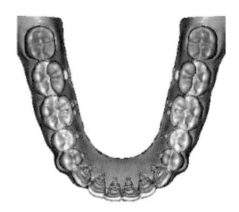

Her treatment plan was to reduce crowding with interproximal reduction, use comprehensive orthodontics to reduce the maxillary protrusion, and above all keep her occlusal trauma to a minimum so that we would not aggravate her recently corrected temporomandibular dysfunction.

I designed a broader arch form to minimize the damage that may result from the interproximal reduction. I did not want to cause any recession as I developed my arch form.

The bracket design on the lower arch incorporates a self-ligation slot to help reduce crowding. Given that there is a lot of crowding, it is likely that all of the teeth would not be tied in from the first visit. This helps to prevent flaring out of the lower incisors and loss of crown torque. The bracket design incorporated half occlusal pads to permanently open the patient's occlusion while we are in treatment. This design not only allows me to remove her nighttime occlusal splint but also to keep the plunging cusp tips of the teeth in crossbite from occluding and preventing tooth movement and the correction of the crossbite.

The prescription called for 0.8 mm of IPR across the lower incisors.

I let the patient know that I felt her teeth would not move any farther forward than

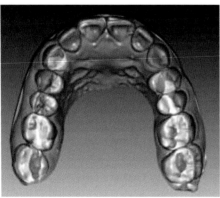
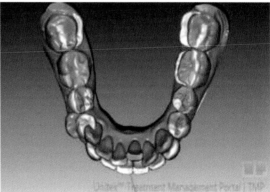

they already had. We planned to look at our progress in 6–9 months' time, to see whether further IPR would be required to reduce dental protrusion further. The case treated out as follows.

Initial presentation of the Class I malocclusion with a unilateral crossbite

Completed correction in 14 months of comprehensive treatment.

The above images indicate the starting position of the lower teeth. The middle image shows how the wire starts in the self-ligation slot to build transverse width into the arch. Note how not all of the teeth are

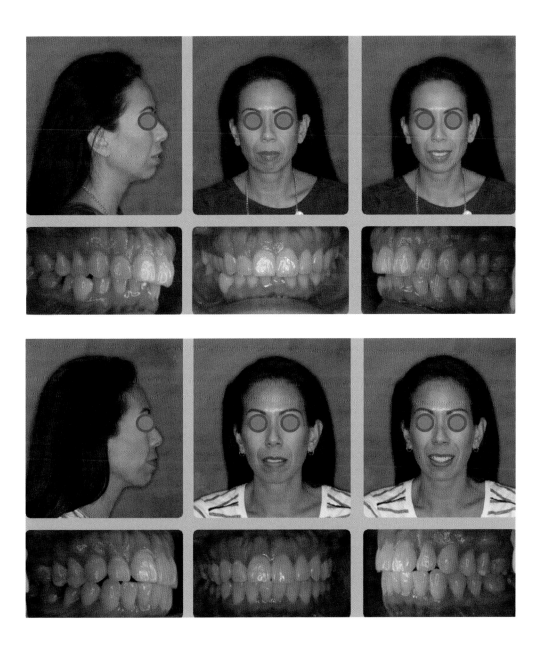

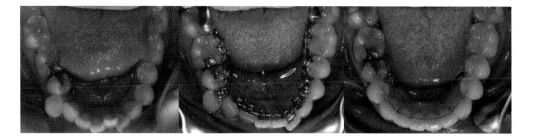

engaged fully to prevent flaring of the lower incisors.

The final results speak for themselves. As predicted in TMP, our results resolved the crossbite and did not cause any periodontal recession.

In conclusion, the Incognito appliance system is an excellent tool to correct any malocclusion, regardless of its severity. It utilizes state-of-the-art technology to setup predictive modeling, which is used to reverse engineer custom brackets and wires. In the future as technology improves, it is reasonable to think that more systems will take this symbiotic approach to customize orthodontic appliances, being respectful of the presenting physiology.

Part 2: eBrace and eLock Lingual Appliances

Thomas W. Örtendahl and K. Hero Breuning

Short history

The customized lingual bracket eBrace is a system which was developed in December 2008 in China by the Guangzhou Riton Biomaterial Company based in the Guangzhou International Biotech Island, Guangdong, China. In August 2009, the first clinical trial with the eBrace appliance started. this system has been tested at several universities in China. This custom system for lingual orthodontic appliance has now applied for several national and international patents. The system has an ISO certificate and is also US FDA approved. The self-ligating version of the system (eLock) is an alternative lingual bracket made by the same company. After the initial introduction of the self-ligating bracket in 2010, the "III generation eBrace III and the eLock II bracket" were introduced in 2015.

Workflow for eBrace and eLock

If the initial treatment plan is to use custom lingual orthodontic appliances, the traditional indirect method of making an impression of the upper and lower dentition with silicone impression material (PVS) can be used to copy the dentition. These impressions and a bite registration can then be sent to the Guangzhou Riton Biomaterial Company in China by UPS or DHL in Europe and FedEx in the US. The company also accepts STL files from scanned dental models or PVS impressions. Of course, intraoral scanners—such as the iTero scanner, Lava scanner, Trios scanner (3Shape), the True Definition scanner, and other intraoral scanners—can be used to scan the dentition and the occlusion directly. It is possible to send all the documentation (e.g. STL files of the dentition, digital photographs including intra- and extraoral images and 2D or radiographs such as an OPT and headplate or a CBCT radiographic image) for a specific patient to the company using large-file services such as "You Send It" or the files can be by uploaded via the secure FTP server. If the orthodontist uses dedicated software such as Ortho-Analyser by 3Shape, STL files of a DSL made in the orthodontic office can be send to the company for appliance fabrication with the 3Shape communicating system. Depending on the orders from the orthodontist, the STL files can be transformed in the orthodontic office or by the lab technicians of the Guangzhou Riton Biomaterial Company using specific software into digital dental models. These digital dental models can then be transferred via the Internet to the office where the orthodontist can analyze the case (measurements of the dentition, Bolton analysis etc.) with orthodontic analyzing software such as Ortho-Analyser and 3M or the Guangzhou Riton Biomaterial Company's software. When the orthodontist has finished treatment planning, this treatment plan will be discussed with the patient. If the treatment plan has been accepted by the patient and fixed lingual orthodontic appliances are selected for the actual treatment, the web-based online ordering and submission platform prescription sheet can be filled in on the company's website

If a traditional setup with plaster and wax is selected, the pictures of the setup will be transferred as a pdf file to the practitioner. This file can be reviewed with a viewer. Changes in the setup have to be indicated by the practitioner. When the setup is approved by the orthodontist, the company should receive an acknowledgement.

For the fabrication of each lingual custom appliance system, a specific lab order form has to be filled in.

The design of the brackets starts with the bracket base. The outline of the custom bracket base and the mesh pad of the custom lingual bracket will be designed according to the preferences of the orthodontist, which should be indicated on the lab's order file. The mesh pad of lingual custom brackets will be usually designed as large as possible to allow reliable bonding to the dentition. Because of the individual design of the bracket base includes occlusal rests for premolars and molars, fewer bracket failures can be expected (Figure 11.1).

Of course, it is essential to select an optimal bracket and tube configuration for each individual treatment. The orthodontist can select different bracket configurations for a custom lingual bracket system: a bracket system with eBrace III brackets (traditional ligating with ligatures and elastic modules) can be ordered with a slot size dimension of $0.018'' \times 0.025''$ (Figure 11.2).

For the cuspid and incisor region, the slot of the lingual bracket can be positioned in a vertical or horizontal direction, depending on the orthodontist's preferences (Figure 11.3).

According to frequent users of lingual appliances, a horizontal position of the slot will result in a nice angulation and tip control, but with reduced rotational control. A vertical position of the bracket slot will improve torque correction. The horizontal position of

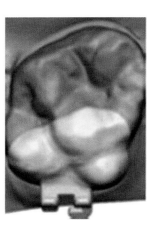 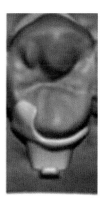

Figure 11.1 Design of occlusal rests for premolars and molars.

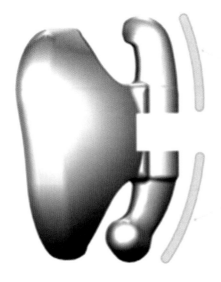

Figure 11.2 Design of the eBrace III brackets.

the slot enables easier sliding of the teeth in the desired direction.

A horizontal slot in the cuspid and incisor region can be helpful in cases where opening a space in the arch is required for implant placement. A vertical slot position can be more efficient to correct the incisor torque, for instance in Class II cases. Optimal tip and torque correction can be achieved in the finishing phase of treatment if full-size finishing wires are used.

A second bracket selection option is to select self-ligating lingual brackets eLock II brackets (Figure 11.4).

Advantages of these self-ligating custom brackets are: easier and faster wire changes and optimal settling of the wires in the bracket slot. Using eLock brackets improves the sliding of teeth along the wire, without reduction of torque and rotational control. This bracket could be the bracket of choice in cases where space should be created for an implant in the frontal region. In non-customized or traditional systems for lingual orthodontic treatment, side effects caused by standard brackets or poor ligation during space closure can be expected. The design of the eLock brackets also helps the orthodontist to maintain or correct the angulation of teeth. For eLock brackets, there is no need for power ties.

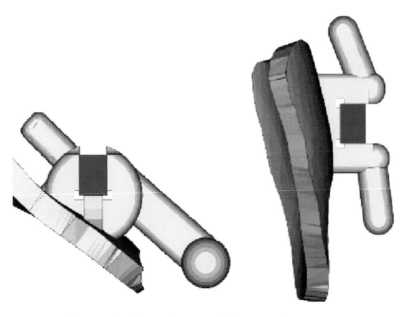

Figure 11.3 A horizontal and vertical position of the slot can be selected.

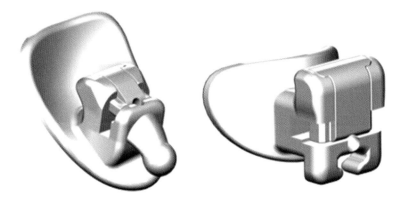

Figure 11.4 Design of self-ligating lingual eLock II brackets.

eBrace or eLock lingual brackets?

The use of custom self-ligating lingual eLock brackets for lingual treatment compared to traditional ligation of the wire to the eBrace bracket has some advantages. The faster change of wires will be less physically demanding for the orthodontist or the dental assistant. A second advantage of self-ligating lingual brackets is there will be no need to check the positioning of the wire in the bracket slot as should be done for treatment with eBrace brackets. Only when the wire is completely seated in the eLock bracket slot can the clip be closed (a clicking sound will be heard). The clips in this eLock system are made from NiCr or Co-Cr and will normally not break. If eLock brackets are selected and a clip should break, all kinds of ligatures used in eBrace lingual brackets can be used to finish the case. Of course a replacement bracket can also be ordered.

Disadvantages of the self-ligating lingual brackets are: a more expensive bracket and wider mesial distal dimension of the bracket. This larger dimension of the brackets will reduce the inter-bracket distance and will cause more bracket interferences at the beginning of the treatment. If interference of the brackets owing to severe crowding or rotation of teeth occurs, or if the total correction of a tooth position cannot be accomplished with one lingual bracket, the technician will design a second (eBrace) bracket ("transitional bracket") that can be used during the early phases of treatment. After partial control of the tooth position, a second bracket will be placed for finishing treatment (Figure 11.5).

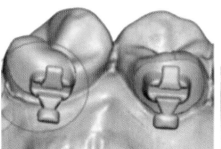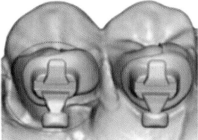

Figure 11.5 A second bracket will be placed for finishing treatment.

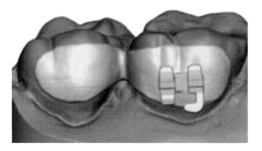

Figure 11.6 A combined mesh pad to improve the stability of the dentition.

Usually, transitional lingual brackets can be needed for lower cuspids and upper lateral incisors and for severely rotated teeth. The technician will decide which tooth should have transitional brackets. However, when the orthodontist evaluates the set-up and decides that a transitional bracket is needed, an extra bracket can be ordered, without extra costs.

As in some cases, the position of the second molars should be stabilized. In those cases a combined mesh pad for the first and second molar can be ordered to increase the stability of the dentition and improve the comfort of the patient (Figure 11.6).

For eBrace and eLock bands, no separation is needed, because the contact points of the molars normally will not be included in the band design (Figure 11.7). Palatal sheets for removable transpalatal arches (TPA or

Goshgarian) or a fixed palatal arch can be ordered. The need for buccal headgear tubes for a Class II corrector, such as Forcus springs and Jasper Jumpers, should be indicated on the prescription sheet. A band on lower premolars including an attachment for Herbst appliances can be indicated on the prescription sheet. If needed, the company can make a (provisional) crown or provisional bridges to be used during treatment.

Occlusal pads on premolars and molars will be used to reduce bracket failures and to enable accurate bonding and rebonding of these brackets. The outline of the occlusal pad for premolars and molars should be indicated on the prescription sheet. Selective coverage (only distal coverage) of the occlusal pad, to reduce the visibility of the appliance, can be selected. For all brackets, the coverage of teeth will act as a bite raiser. It is recommended to order onlays only for premolars in the lower dentition as other onlays will interfere with the adaptation of the occlusion.

To effectively open the occlusion, horizontal stops on incisor and cuspid brackets (bite raisers) can be ordered. However, we prefer to use acrylic buildups to unlock the occlusion for most cases. The design of the brackets will reduce tongue irritation (Figure 11.8a–c). If required, buccal tubes for molars can be ordered (Figure 11.9).

For the eBrace and eLock appliances, different appliance materials (NiCr, Co-Cr, or

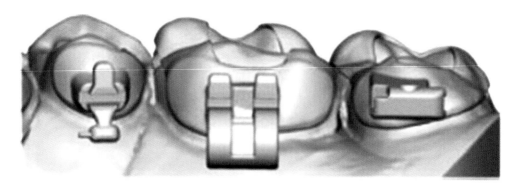

Figure 11.7 The contact points of the molars normally will not be included.

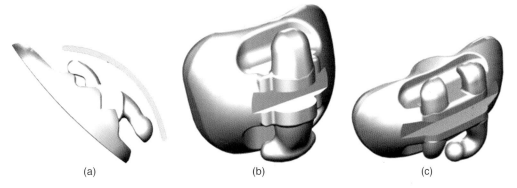

(a) (b) (c)

Figure 11.8 (a–c) The design of the brackets will reduce tongue irritation.

gold) can be selected. After the removal of the braces used, eBrace brackets can be sent to the company for recycling. For eLock appliances, gold cannot be selected as an option.

The bracket base of the custom brackets has no mesh pad and has a permanent marking for bracket identification. The pads are ready for bonding; no primer or sandblasting is needed.

The hooks on all eBrace and eLock brackets can be used for interarch elastic placement.

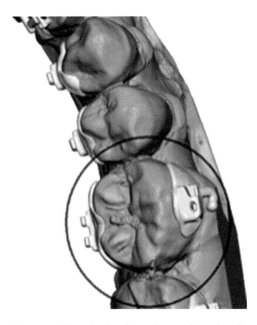

Figure 11.9 Buccal tubes for molars can be ordered.

Power chain can be easily placed over the wires and will remain on each bracket. If eLock brackets are selected, nickel titanium (NiTi) push coil as well as NiTi retraction coils can be used without side effects.

Wires for eBrace and eLock brackets

The custom orthodontic wires should closely fit in the bracket slot and will move the teeth in the desired direction. The diameter and flexibility of the wires can be ordered depending on the preferences of the orthodontist. For both systems, a selection of wires can be ordered: usually a set of five wires will be sufficient to treat a case. For the upper and lower incisal brackets, a self-ligation option is available (Figure 11.10).

Extra wires can be chosen but there will be a fee for these extra wires. Traditional mushroom shape arc forms can be used for lingual treatment.

The custom bracket will then be rather "bulky." To reduce the thickness of the brackets (which will increase patient comfort), bending of the wire can be simulated. For optimal reduction of the thickness of the brackets, a wire with more bends can be designed. Custom wires ordered for this custom lingual system will usually have only horizontal corrections (Figure 11.11). In extraction cases, a specific part of the wire should be straight to allow space closure. The

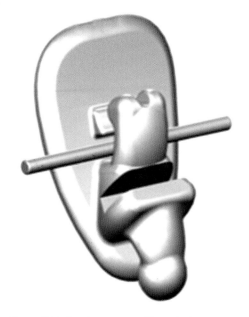

Figure 11.10 For the upper and lower incisors a self-ligation slot can be used.

advantage of using wires with only horizontal corrections to reduce the distance between the bracket base and bracket slot is a better fit of the wire in the bracket slot, as there is no torque and tip in the wires. All the custom torque and tip corrections needed will be designed into the bracket slot. If required, wires with extra (10 degrees) torque can be ordered to compensate for the treatment mechanics (e.g. Class II elastics) used. If indicated, a final arch with increased or reduced width can be ordered to correct extreme narrow or extreme wide arches. We strongly suggest finishing each eBrace and eLock case with full-size stainless steel or TMA wires. These finishing wires will reduce the need for wires with extra torque or arch compensation. Because this system will use only flat wires, changing the wires will be easier compared to some other systems. If there is a need to replace a broken steel or TMA wire due to

Figure 11.11 The custom wires will usually have only horizontal corrections.

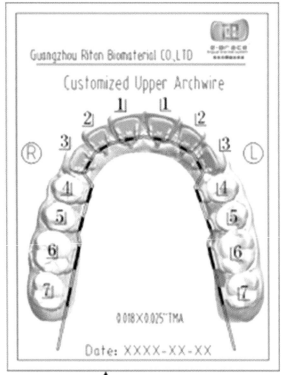

fracture, it is even possible to bend this wire yourself, or you can order a spare custom-made wire.

Setup for a specific case

The company's orthodontic lab will make a dental setup according to the treatment plan and prescription formulas that were uploaded by the orthodontist.

For this setup, a traditional setup in plaster and wax or a digital dental setup can be chosen. After finalization of the manual or DSL, a pdf file of the setup will be sent to the office of the orthodontist by mail.

For the DSL, the accuracy of the provided digital dental model will be evaluated; for lingual appliances, the impression of the lingual surface should be optimal. If the quality of the impression is not sufficient for appliance fabrication, the orthodontist will receive an email and will be asked to send in another impression.

The eBrace and eLock company now use both the Ortho-Analyser (3Shape) software and their own software to make a digital dental setup. So, if the orthodontist has the Ortho-Analyser program, and uses a desktop impression or plaster model scanner or an intraoral scanner to get a digital dental model, the orthodontist could make the setup with the Ortho-Analyser software and send the files with Communicator (3Shape, Denmark) to the Guangzhou Riton Biomaterial Company. The technician will review each case's documentation and treatment plan provided by the orthodontist. If during the fabrication of a setup there is any doubt the planned movements will be possible, the orthodontist will receive an email to discuss this suggested treatment plan. The amount and location of interproximal reduction needed for a specific setup will be indicated by the software. Communication with the technical lab for eBrace and eLock cases will not be a problem, as a technician will be available 24 hours a day, seven days a week to discuss a case. There will also always be someone available who speaks English. Of course, it is important that the orthodontist answers every query regarding a specific patient. If the company does not receive a returning mail after sending a setup, completion of this specific case will be stopped after a few days until a proper reaction is received.

At the moment, it is only possible to review the original and planned digital dental model in all directions, using a 3D viewer, unless the orthodontist has the Ortho-Analyser software. Superimposition of the dental model before and after treatment using this pdf file and of course with the 3Shape software is possible. If the 3D viewer is used, the orthodontist has to indicate changes to be made in the setup in the responding email. The company expects the orthodontist to provide software for their customers, which can be used to analyze the digital dental model (make measurements on the models) for treatment planning and to allow the orthodontist to correct the suggested setup according to his/her personal wishes. Limited correction of a setup by the technical lab will be included in the total fee, but major changes to a treatment plan (e.g. a change from non-extraction to extraction) will be charged by the company.

Indirect bonding of custom lingual appliances

A selection of indirect bonding trays and jigs can be chosen. For incisors and cuspids, acrylic positioning jigs are available.

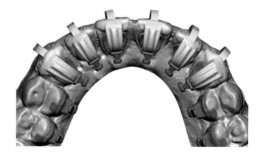

Figure 11.12 Rebonding jigs for the lingual custom brackets.

Silicone or transparent indirect bonding trays for full arch bonding can also be ordered. For incisal and cuspid brackets, repositioning jigs are virtually designed and these jigs can be printed to be used for accurate rebonding (Figure 11.12).

Further reading for Parts 1 and 2

Auluck, A. (2013) Lingual orthodontic treatment: what is the current evidence base? *J. Orthod.*, **40** (suppl. 1), S27–S33.

Barthelemi, S., Hyppolite, M.P., Palot, C., and Wiechmann D. (2014) Components of overbite correction in lingual orthodontics: molar extrusion or incisor intrusion? *Int. Orthod.*, **12** (4), 395–412.

Dalessandri, D., Lazzaroni, E., Migliorati, M., *et al.* (2013) Self-ligating fully customized lingual appliance and chair-time reduction: a typodont study followed by a randomized clinical trial. *Eur. J. Orthod.*, **35** (6), 758–765.

Galletti, C., Fauquet-Roure, C., and Raybaud, P. (2010) Treatment of Class III malocclusions in adults using the Incognito® lingual technique. *Int. Orthod.*, **8** (3), 227–252.

Grauer, D. and Proffit, W.R. (2011) Accuracy in tooth positioning with a fully customized lingual orthodontic appliance. *Am. J. Orthod. Dentofacial Orthop.*, **140** (3), 433–443.

Grauer, D., Wiechmann, D., Heymann, G.C., and Swift, E.J. Jr. (2012) Computer-aided design/computer-aided manufacturing technology in customized orthodontic appliances. *J. Esthet. Restor. Dent.*, **24** (1), 3–9.

Huntley, P.N. (2013) Avoiding pitfalls in planning with the Incognito lingual system. *J Orthod.*, **40** (suppl. 1), S54–S9.

Hutchinson, I. and Lee, J.Y. (2013) Fabrication of lingual orthodontic appliances: past, present and future. *J. Orthod.*, **40** (suppl. 1), S14–S9.

Knösel, M., Klang, E., Helms, H.J., and Wiechmann, D. (2014) Lingual orthodontic treatment duration: performance of two different completely customized multi-bracket appliances (Incognito and WIN) in groups with different treatment complexities. *Head Face Med.*, **1** (10), 46.

Kwon, S.Y., Kim, Y., Ahn, H.W., *et al.* (2014) Computer-aided designing and manufacturing of lingual fixed orthodontic appliance using 2D/3D registration software and rapid prototyping. *Int. J. Dent.*, doi: 10.1155/2014/164164.

Lawson, R.B. (2013) Class II correction with the Incognito lingual appliance. *J. Orthod.*, **40** (suppl. 1), S49–S53.

Lawson, R.B. (2013) Extraction treatment in lingual orthodontics. *J. Orthod.*, **40** (suppl. 1), S38–S48.

Sifakakis, I., Pandis, N., Makou, M., *et al.* (2013) A comparative assessment of torque generated by lingual and conventional brackets. *Eur. J. Orthod.*, **35** (3), 375–380.

Sifakakis, I., Pandis, N., Makou, M., *et al.* (2013) A comparative assessment of forces and moments generated by lingual and conventional brackets. *Eur. J. Orthod.*, **35** (1), 82–86.

Wiechmann, D., Klang, E., Helms, H.J., and Knösel, M. (2015) Lingual appliances reduce the incidence of white spot lesions during orthodontic multibracket treatment. *Am. J. Orthod. Dentofacial. Orthop.*, **148** (3), 414–422.

Wiechmann, D., Gerss, J., Stamm, T., and Hohoff, A. (2008) Prediction of oral discomfort and dysfunction in lingual orthodontics: a preliminary report. *Am. J. Orthod. Dentofacial Orthop.*, **133** (3), 359–364.

Zinelis, S., Sifakakis, I., Katsaros, C., and Eliades, T. (2014) Microstructural and mechanical characterization of contemporary lingual orthodontic brackets. *Eur. J. Orthod.*, **36** (4), 389–393.

Part 3: Harmony Appliance Systems

Chung H. Kau and K. Hero Breuning

Lingual appliances have made tremendous progress since their first inception by Fujita in 1979 [1, 2]. The methods of manufacturing, appliance design, and biomechanical therapy have improved greatly over the last two decades [3–5]. Patients ask or even demand less visible orthodontic appliances. As aligner therapy is still not indicated for the full range of orthodontic malocclusions and only a limited part of the orthodontist has been trained to treat patients with aligners, the alternative of lingual fixed appliances is an option to meet the wishes of patients. There are advantages to lingual appliances, and not only because of their improved esthetics: lingual fixed appliances can be used for better white spot lesion control and there is better anchorage control with palatal placed microscrew implants [6, 7]. These factors have made lingual appliances more accepted in the orthodontic marketplace.

Traditional appliances

Lingual appliances are not easy appliances to construct, because of the individual shape of the dentition on the lingual surfaces. The actual laboratory fabrication of the custom-made lingual appliance requires a tremendous amount of skill and precision. The design of lingual brackets and the fabrication of this design with the use of three-dimensional (3D) printers is tedious and time-consuming, often requiring advanced dental laboratory knowledge translated from the documentation and treatment plan provided by the orthodontist into the clinical environment of orthodontic appliance fabrication.

Description of the Harmony appliance

The original appliance was invented by Dr. Patrick Curiel (an orthodontist working in Paris) and Philippe Salah (a computer technician) and was, after a test period in France and Europe, acquired by American Orthodontics [8]. At that time and to date, the system combines the latest computer-aided design and computer-aided manufacturing (CAD/CAM) processes and manufacturing techniques to meet the most stringent clinical requirements in the industry. The Harmony appliance is the first system in the world to have:

1. a digital laboratory workflow;
2. robotically formed arch wires;
3. interactive self-ligating brackets;
4. customized 3D printed bonding pads;
5. anterior re-positioning jigs;
6. digitally assisted treatment monitoring;
7. deliverance of progress setups and progress wires.

Digital laboratory workflow

The main stages of the laboratory process for all custom lingual appliances are as follows. First, a high-quality dental impression or intraoral scan is taken. The impressions are often done in polyvinyl siloxane (PVS) material after which a high-quality representation of the dentition is poured into stone. Almost always, a duplicate malocclusion study cast is made. In a traditional workflow with plaster casts, the dental casts are mounted in a semi-adjusted dental articulator that replicates or represents the range of motion of the jaw. Next, the dental cast is carefully sectioned so that the teeth may be individually set up to an ideal and esthetic occlusion. The articulator can be used to maintain the original occlusal plane.

For custom lingual appliance systems, such as Harmony and eBrace/eLock, only digital dental models are used. The use of digital models facilitates the transfer of the dental model and can be used to make custom appliances based on a virtual setup. These models also facilitate orthodontic analysis and allow visualization of the orthodontic treatment planning before the actual decision to order a specific appliance (such as custom fixed appliances or aligners). The procedure of making a virtual setup for diagnostic purposes or the fabrication of custom orthodontic appliances, compared to the traditional method in plaster and wax, is less time consuming. Setup accuracy can be improved if digital dental models are used, because a possible loss in the tooth structure during the cutting process of the plaster will be avoided during the digital dental crown separation procedure.

The segmentation techniques for dental crowns depend on the specific software used. In a virtual setup, dental movement simulating an orthodontic treatment can be quantified and visualized in all directions, and can be easily redone when required. For each case, dental arch expansion, reduction of interdental tooth material ("stripping"), or the decision to extract teeth can be evaluated.

It is important to mention that on computers tooth movements are unlimited. Teeth alignment and levelling can be designed on the computer screen, but this planned result by a lab technician may not be realistic for that specific patient.

A virtual dental setup can be used to virtually design buccal as well as lingual brackets.

Robotically formed arch wires

Large variations in the lingual surface of teeth do not allow a pre-adjusted system to be available for lingual appliances (Figure 11.13).

As a result, all of the positions of the custom brackets for custom lingual systems, such as Harmony, are dictated by the arch wire designed on the virtual setup of the dentition. Robotically formed arch wires as used in the Harmony system give the system much precision especially in maintaining and obtaining the final arch form. The gradual buildup of the robotic arch wire sequence allows for lighter forces to be delivered to teeth. However, the biggest advantage is close adaptability of the wire to the lingual surface of the teeth. This finishing wire, the "master wire," is used to dictate the bracket positions of individual teeth on the malocclusion model. For the Harmony system, the master wire comes in three forms: straight wire, a traditional pre-adjusted arch form, or a mushroom-shaped arch. The compensation for the distance between the wire and the lingual tooth surface is made in the 3D-printed metal mesh pad which fills in the distance between the lingual surfaces and the self-ligating lingual brackets and tubes. Hence, when traditional mushroom wires are used, there is a significant amount of bulkiness to the brackets. Alternative wires can be selected and, depending on the wire shape selected, there is greater adaptability of the arch wire to the lingual surface of the tooth. If an optimal adaptability of the arch wire to the lingual surface of the tooth is selected, a significant amount of wire bending by the computer is required and the best fit between the wire and the tooth surface can be achieved. Harmony offers the possibility to select

Figure 11.13 Design of custom bonding pads.
Company: American Orthodontics.

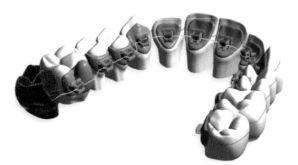

an "optimized archform." If this option is selected, the amount of wire bending is reduced, and the bulkiness of the brackets will be acceptable. Of course, the wire shape should be corrected for extraction cases. The shape of this master wire is then used for a series of wires of different dimensions and flexibility to be used during treatment.

Interactive self-ligating brackets

Lingual brackets have two tie wings (occlusal and gingival placed). This design allows the bracket to be smaller in size and a decreased inter-bracket distance. This is important, as the interbracket distance for lingual brackets is always reduced compared to buccally placed brackets. The drawback of this design means that the clinician needs to be technically proficient to ligate the bracket during the arch wire bracket interface. The chairside time therefore increases considerably for lingual appliances and so does the technical skill of the orthodontist. This underlying factor has been one of the biggest drawbacks of orthodontists wanting to practice lingual orthodontics. Probably the biggest advantage of the Harmony system is that it possesses a self-ligating clip (Figure 11.14). This revolution in technology has lowered the threshold

for orthodontists wanting to get involved in lingual appliances. The ability to fully create an effective and efficient arch wire/bracket interface using the clip now means that elaborate ligation ties with metal ligatures or elastic rings are no longer necessary. The downside of the large clip needed to have sufficient control over the wire/bracket contact is that the reduction of the inter-bracket distance between two teeth. However, the ease of ligating the arch wire far outweighs the loss of inter-bracket distance.

The introduction of self-ligating custom lingual appliances enables the relatively fast removal and engagement of wires and the use of low forces, less friction, easy sliding, and the use of push coils for lingual treatment. Practitioners who selected self-ligating bracket systems for buccal treatment do not need to select traditional ligation for lingual treatment but can use the same system for lingual treatment.

Customized bonding pads

The digital set-up has allowed customized pads to be fabricated for the system (Figure 11.13). In a routine setup, computer modeling is applied to aid in the design of the bonding pads. This allows better adaptability and also the engineering to create the best surface area for the pad to adapt to the tooth. This maximizes the bonding surface area and enhances the bond strength of the bracket (Figure 11.14). Once the design of the pad has been accomplished, a customized connector is fabricated to minimize the physical size of the bracket.

Anterior positioning jigs

Normally, the brackets are embedded within a transfer tray to aid the transfer of the bracket to the dentition. In some cases, it is not possible to bond all teeth in one session, owing to the amount of crowding or

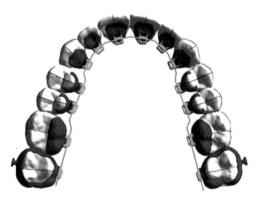

Figure 11.14 Occlusal bonding pads, for stability and bite raising.
Company: American Orthodontics.

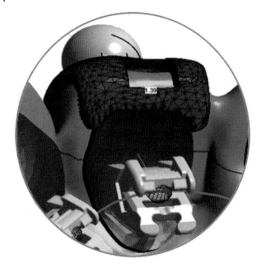

Figure 11.15 Design of rebonding jigs.
Company: American Orthodontics.

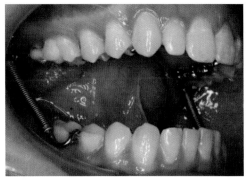

Figure 11.16 Forsus spring in combination with Harmony.
Company: 3M and American Orthodontists.

uneruption. For the Harmony system, anterior positioning jigs are provided for all incisors and cuspids to allow the orthodontist to bond select teeth at a later date (Figure 11.15). These jigs are also especially useful in situations when debonding of the bracket has occurred.

Digitally assisted treatment

As with all digital setups the ability to manipulate and visualize the treatment helps clinicians to diagnose, plan, and anticipate problems in the treatment process and final setup. During treatment, a progress impression or a progress intraoral scan can be used to evaluate the treatment progress. If needed, a progress setup can be made and progress wires can be ordered to finish the individual case according to the original treatment plan. If needed, elastics and Class II correction springs such as Forsus springs can be used during treatment (Figure 11.16).

Discussions

A recent published systematic review showed that lingual appliances were associated with

overall oral discomfort compared with labial appliances [9]. In addition, lingual appliances were also associated with an increase in speech impediment. It has been shown that speech disturbances are associated with bracket design and could be a greater embarrassment than visible labial brackets. This has made the actual design of the bracket so much more important. Alternative systems with only a customized base made with bonding material are more bulky compared to the customized lingual appliance systems, such as Incognito, Harmony, and eBrace/eLock.

In the literature, it was mentioned that a change of the intercanine width (expansion) is another drawback of lingual appliances [10]. It was concluded that most lingual cases increase the intercanine width. Digital customization allows for meticulous planning and results in an arch shape that is more predictable. In addition, the use of robotic wires helps to limit unwanted expansion (Figure 11.17).

One of the main problems with lingual systems is that wire bending for lingual cases to create the intricate first-, second-, and third-order bends is more challenging. But as intraoral scanning during treatment will become more incorporated in the workflow for orthodontics, it will become easier to ask for progress and follow up finishing wires for lingual cases. This use of progress wires can

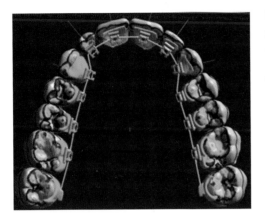

Figure 11.17 Design for custom lingual wires.
Company: American Orthodontics.

be used to correct unplanned side effects during treatment and thus stimulate fast and efficient treatment with lingual cases.

Conclusion

The Harmony system is a revolutionary new system that incorporates many advantages of the digital era. The incorporation of the self-ligating bracket and the robotic bended wires has made lingual orthodontics a real alternative for less esthetic orthodontic appliances and is now a successful alternative in modern orthodontics.

References

1 Fujita, K. (1982) Multilingual-bracket and mushroom arch wire technique: a clinical report. *Am. J. Orthod.*, **82**, 120–140.

2 Fujita, K. (1979) New orthodontic treatment with lingual bracket mushroom arch wire appliance. *Am. J. Orthod.*, **76**, 657–675.

3 Hutchinson, I. and Lee, J.Y. (2013) Fabrication of lingual orthodontic appliances: past, present and future. *J. Orthod.*, **40** (suppl. 1), S14–S19.

4 Ye, L. and Kula, K.S. (2006) Status of lingual orthodontics. *World J. Orthod.*, **7**, 361–368.

5 Sharif, M.O., Waring, D., and Malik, O.II. (2015) Lingual orthodontics: the future? *Int. J. Orthod. Milwaukee*, **26**, 49–52.

6 Wilmes, B., Nienkemper, M., Mazaud-Schmelter, M., *et al.* (2013) Combined use of Beneslider and lingual braces, mechanical aspects and procedures. *Orthod. Fr.*, **84**, 347–359.

7 Wiechmann, D., Klang, E., Helms, H.J., and Knösel, M. (2015) Lingual appliances reduce the incidence of white spot lesions during orthodontic multibracket treatment. *Am. J. Orthod. Dentofacial Orthop.*, **148**, 414–422.

8 American Orthodontics (2016) *The Harmony System*, http://www.american ortho.com/harmony.html, accessed November 21, 2016.

9 Long, H., Zhou, Y., Pyakurel, U. *et al.* (2013) Comparison of adverse effects between lingual and labial orthodontic treatment: a systematic review. *Angle Orthodontist*, **83** (6), 1066–1073.

10 Khattab, T.Z., Hajeer, M.Y., Farah, H., and Al-Sabbagh, R.J. (2014) Maxillary dental arch changes following the leveling and alignment stage with lingual and labial orthodontic appliances: a preliminary report of a randomized controlled trial. *Contemp. Dent. Pract.*, **15** (5), 561–566.

Appendix

3D Systems 333 Three D Systems Circle, Rock Hill, SC, USA

3dMD LLC 3200, Cobb Galleria Parkway 203, Atlanta, GA, USA

3M I-94 and McKnight, StPaul, MN, USA

3Shape Headquarters Europe, Middle East & Africa Sales: Holmens Kanal 7, 1060, Copenhagen, Denmark

Align Technology, Inc. 2560 Orchard Parkway, San Jose, CA, USA

American Orthodontics 3524 Washington Avenue P.O. Box 1048 Sheboygan, WI 53081-1048, USA

Anatomage Inc: 111 N. Market St., Suite 500, San Jose, CA, USA

Dental Monitoring 47 Avenue Hoche, 75008, Paris, France

Dolphin Imaging & Management Solutions 9200 Eton Ave., Chatsworth, CA, USA

Exceed-Ortho Roosikrantsi 2 K-120, Tallinn 10119, Estonia

Great Lakes Orthodontics 200 Cooper Avenue, Tonawanda, NY, USA

Guangzhou Riton Biomaterial Co Unit 101–103, Floor 1, Research District A and B, Luo Xuan Road, 3 Gangzhou, International Bioisland, China

Image Instruments Olbernhauer Str. 5, 09125 Chemnitz, Germany

Kerr Corporation Via Strecce 4, PO BOX 268, 6934 Bioggio, Switzerland

Medicim Company Stationsstraat 102, b6–2800 Mechelen, Belgium

Memotain 10 Willettstraße, 40822 Mettmann, Germany

Opal Orthodontics 505 West, 10200 South, South Jordan, UT, USA

OraMetrix 2350 Campbell Creek Blvd, Suite 400, Richardson, TX, USA

Ormco 1717 West Collins, Orange, CA, USA

Ortho Caps GmbH 8An der Bewer, 59069 Hamm, Germany

Ortholab 8 Dorpsplein, 3941JH, Doorn, the Netherlands

Orthoproof 8-C Edisonbaan, 3439 MN Nieuwegein, the Netherlands

Digital Planning and Custom Orthodontic Treatment, First Edition. Edited by K. Hero Breuning and Chung H. Kau.
© 2017 John Wiley & Sons, Inc. Published 2017 by John Wiley & Sons, Inc.

Planmeca Oy Asentajankatu 6, FIN-00880, Helsinki, Finland

Sirona Dental Systems GmbH Fabrikstraße 31D-64625 Bensheim, Germany

suresmile 2350 Campbell Creek Blvd, Suite 400, Richardson, TX, USA

TOP-Service für Lingualtechnik GmbH 81Schledehauser Straße, 49152 Bad Essen, Germany

Index

3dMD   28–29
3Shape   2, 57–58

a
ALARA   2
aligners   42, 47, 70
Anatomage   10

c
CAD/CAM   41, 47, 66, 68
Carestream Dental   58
ClinCheck   70, 76
Cloud   13, 31
computerized planning   45
Cone Beam Technology (CBCT)   2, 9, 29
custom appliance design   41, 44
custom retention   65
custom wire   49

d
dental models   29
dental monitoring   56–62
DICOM   10
digital assisted treatment   112
digital work flow   39
Dolphin   10, 58, 63
dynamic motion   15

e
eBrace/eLock   45, 49

Emiluma   49
exceed software   49

f
field of view (FOV)   9–10, 12
file transfer protocol (FTP)   31
FusionBite Tray   16

g
Geomagic   6

h
Harmony system   44, 109–113
Herbst   41

i
Incognito   44, 83–85
indirect bonding trays   44
Insignia   35
intra-oral scanner   2
intra-oral scans   5
Invisalign   42, 69
iTero   4, 58

j
jaw motion tracking (JMT)   16

k
Kesling setup   31

l
Lumaloc   49

m
mandibular movements   20–25
mandibular repositioning devices   65
Maxillim   6, 63
Memotain retainer   67–68
monitoring tooth movement   55

n
Nola System   50

o
Objective Grading Scale   69
OnyxCeph   43
Opal Orthodontics   49
OraMetrix   28, 43–44
Orchestrate   43
Ortho-Analyzer   27, 33–34, 63
Orthoproof   48

p
Planmeca   28
polyvinyl siloxane (PVS)   35
positioners   65

r
rebonding jig   52
Romexis software   28

s
sandblasting   52
scout view   10

Digital Planning and Custom Orthodontic Treatment, First Edition. Edited by K. Hero Breuning and Chung H. Kau.
© 2017 John Wiley & Sons, Inc. Published 2017 by John Wiley & Sons, Inc.

segmentation (airway) 11, 32
segmentation (crowns) 32
Segmented fixed appliances 74
SiCAT 16
Sirona 16
smartphone 60

stereolithographic files (STL) 2, 5, 27, 67
superimposition 13
suresmile 37

t
T-attachment 16
temporomandibular joint (TMJ) 16

tracking system 15–16
Trios scanner 58

v
virtual arch wire 34
virtual articulator 29
virtual brackets 43
virtual head 27